T0271626

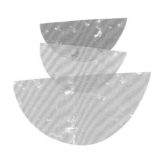

FEED YOUR FAMILY
DAIRY FREE

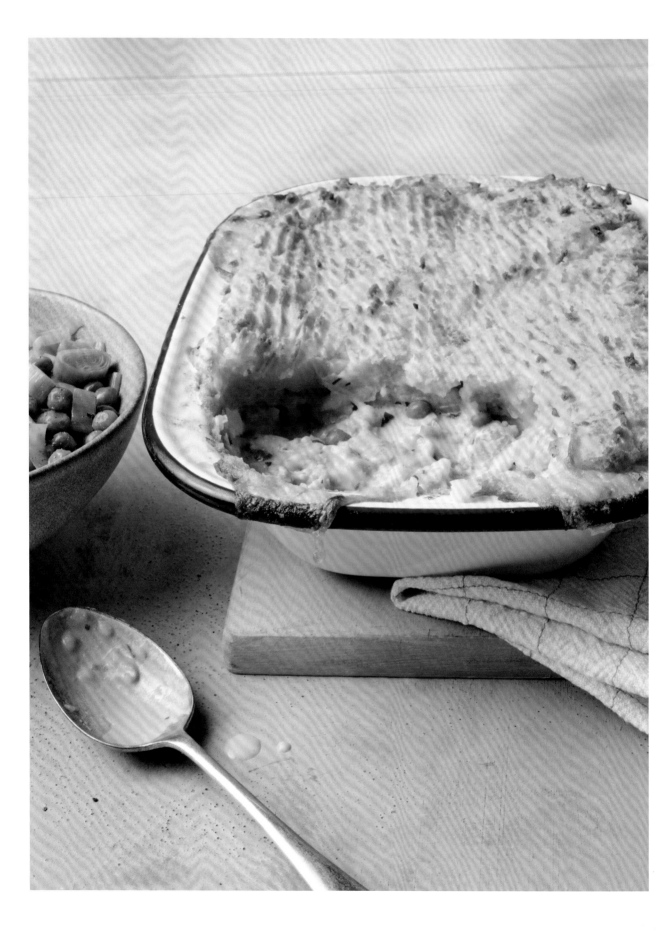

FEED YOUR FAMILY
DAIRY FREE

Weaning + Nutrition + Recipes + Allergy Advice

Kate Lancaster
aka The Dairy Free Mum

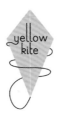

yellow kite

First published in Great Britain in 2024 by Yellow Kite
An imprint of Hodder & Stoughton
An Hachette UK company

1

Copyright © Kate Lancaster 2024
Photography by Jen Rich © Hodder & Stoughton 2024,
except photos on pages 24 and 27 © Rachel
@allergy_mummaandbubba 2024

The right of Kate Lancaster to be identified as the Author
of the Work has been asserted by her in accordance with
the Copyright, Designs and Patents Act 1988.

All rights reserved. No part of this publication may be
reproduced, stored in a retrieval system, or transmitted,
in any form or by any means without the prior written
permission of the publisher, nor be otherwise circulated in
any form of binding or cover other than that in which it is
published and without a similar condition being imposed
on the subsequent purchaser.

A CIP catalogue record for this title is available from the
British Library

Hardback ISBN 978 1 399 73127 0
eBook ISBN 978 1 399 73128 7

Editorial Director: Nicky Ross
Senior Project Editor: Liv Nightingall
Copyeditor: Vicky Orchard
Nutritionist: Lucy Upton
Designer: Louise Leffler
Photography and styling: Jen Rich
Senior Production Controller: Matt Everett

Colour origination by Alta Image London
Printed and bound in China by C&C Offset Printing Co., Ltd.

Hodder & Stoughton policy is to use papers that are natural,
renewable and recyclable products and made from wood
grown in sustainable forests. The logging and manufacturing
processes are expected to conform to the environmental
regulations of the country of origin.

Yellow Kite
Hodder & Stoughton Ltd
Carmelite House
50 Victoria Embankment
London
EC4Y 0DZ

www.yellowkitebooks.co.uk
www.hodder.co.uk

Disclaimer

The information and references contained herein are for informational purposes only,
and the advice given is generalised. They are designed to support, not replace, any
ongoing individualised medical advice given by a healthcare professional and should
not be construed as the giving of medical advice nor relied upon as a basis for any
decision or action. Readers should always consult their doctor or dietitian before
altering their diet, or that of their child. Any concerns about your child should always
be discussed with an appropriate healthcare professional.

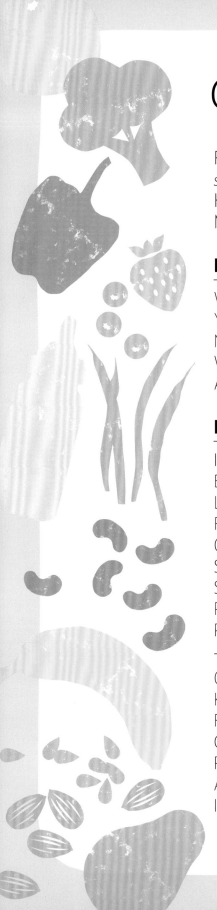

contents

Foreword

By Lucy Upton, specialist paediatric dietitian

As a seasoned paediatric dietitian with over 13 years of experience working with infants and children, and now a mother myself, I can assert with unwavering confidence that nourishing children represents one of the most emotionally charged and demanding, yet ultimately rewarding, daily journeys that parents embark upon. For parents of children with food allergies, or dietary differences, feeding their children has another dimension and is something you simply can't have a day off from!

When I started working with allergy parents, which fortuitously was right from the start of my career, I was compelled to never let this speciality leave my side. I relished the personal challenge of getting to grips with a complex and ever-evolving area of nutrition and health, and there is something about working with parents (and children) with food allergies that has continued to inspire me.

Food allergies knock most parents for six, and understandably so. Without warning, you are thrown into a whirlwind of what I call 'no's and news' - food avoidance, label reading, appointments, nutrition and alternatives. Ultimately a child's feeding journey becomes more complicated, and the feeding mental load triples in size. Even the often joyful aspects of feeding kids - holidays, first birthdays, a summer barbecue with family - are all shrouded with extra vigilance, catering, consideration and often big emotions like fear. Despite this, year in and year out, I have supported families who employ a seemingly endless stream of effort and energy to ensure their children are not just safe, but healthy, happy and thriving in the midst of one or multiple food allergies.

My respect for allergy parents and children alike is also rooted in the fact that food allergies, despite their increasing prevalence, remain a condition relentlessly misunderstood. In a world of health noise, food allergy families continue to find themselves floating amidst a sea of narratives, from being labelled (incorrectly, of course!) as intolerant, to being told they are being overprotective or finding others questioning why they can't even offer 'a little bit'.

Over the last few years, and unfortunately often due to heartbreaking allergy headlines, it feels like public food allergy awareness is finally (albeit slowly) increasing. This is also coupled with rising numbers of children with food allergies, something the World Health Organization now considers to be a 'modern epidemic'. Alongside the work of patient organisations like Allergy UK, there is a community of parents and professionals raising their voices across a multitude of platforms. Amongst this, of course, there is Kate. A mother of two children with food allergies, who has firmly embedded herself as the heart of an online food allergy community, now serving thousands of families. I first 'met' Kate online in the throes of a worldwide pandemic. Her passion and hunger for understanding more about food allergies and advocating for her own children was motivating to say the least. But Kate evidently hasn't stopped at this, she has become an oracle of allergy-friendly food, campaigning fiercely for allergy inclusion but also providing parents with never-ending empathy and understanding.

Across social media, Kate and I have already worked together to support parents by combining my clinical and her parental experience on allergy topics from weaning to the milk ladder, so when Kate approached me about this book, I bit her hand off! This book has been something long missing from the shelves, on a probably overlooked subject - a feeling I know resonates with many allergy families daily. We have strived to bring everything milk-free families need in one place, from evidence-based topics (supported by me) to balanced meals.

On the topic of food, the soul of this book is found in bringing milk-free life alive, with Kate's balanced and vibrant recipes, and not a jacket potato in sight! So many parents come to me desperate for the practical management of a milk-free life, alongside a desire for reassurance that their child is getting everything they need. The meals in this book are that! A beautiful balance of nutritious food your child and family will actually want to eat, paired with the other 'nourishment' food offers - fun, family meals, special occasions and, importantly for the allergy community, inclusivity. This book can be a one-stop shop for so many aspects of food-allergy parenting and dairy-free life. We hope it can provide a lighthouse in what sometimes feels like a dark or murky place for new and seasoned allergy and milk-free families alike.

So, all that remains is for me to express my hope that this book becomes a cherished companion in your home, providing empathetic reassurance and guidance, as well as nourishment and joy. I can confidently say on behalf of both of us that it has been a privilege to contribute to the allergy community's voice, and we are committed to sharing, speaking, and supporting your milk-free family, one page or recipe at a time!

Lucy Upton | www.thechildrensdietitian.co.uk

LUCY UPTON
The
Children's
Dietitian
HEALTH & HAPPINESS

Hi from Kate

A big welcome to *Feed Your Family Dairy Free*! When my eldest child was diagnosed with cow's milk protein allergy (CMPA) and I began my dairy-free journey, I often felt worried, confused and stressed. There were so many times I wished there was a book that could help to guide me. Well, this is that book! Being given the opportunity to write this, and be your companion on your journey, is a real honour. Whether you're a long-time Instagram follower, or new to The Dairy Free Mum, I hope you find it helpful with all my heart.

Being an allergy parent is tough

I'm sending you a hug through this book because I know how anxiety-inducing and overwhelming it can feel to have children with food allergies. It isn't easy, and through my Instagram page, I have spoken to many parents who sadly haven't had the support they desperately need, and have been left feeling lost and helpless.

You may finally have a CMPA diagnosis, only to be told it will be months before an appointment with an allergy clinic or dietitian, and you're stuck thinking 'Well, what do I do now?' You may be approaching weaning, birthdays, holidays or your child starting nursery with dread, worrying about how you can navigate these milestones safely and happily. Perhaps you're concerned about nutrition, unsure how your child will get enough calcium or wondering which plant-based milk alternative is best for them to drink. These are all questions I once asked myself, and the very reason I started The Dairy Free Mum and am now writing this book – to help other allergy parents going through the same experiences.

Dairy free doesn't mean flavour free!

Being told you have to go dairy free can feel daunting. If you're a cheese or chocolate lover, it may even feel impossible! Trust me, I get it. However, I'm here to show you that dairy-free food can be tasty, nutritious and something the whole family can enjoy together.

Some of my favourite messages I receive on social media say things like, 'The kids loved this recipe, and even my dairy-loving partner devoured it – we couldn't believe it was dairy free!' That's exactly the point of the recipes in this book; delicious meals you can all share, so no one has to miss out. I love that we can all eat the same thing at home, so my son Jude doesn't feel excluded, and it reduces my stress levels knowing that he won't grab something from one of our plates that he's not meant to eat. Plus, let's be honest, who has the time or energy to be cooking multiple meals?!

**Being told you have to go dairy free can feel really daunting.
If you're a cheese or chocolate lover, it may even feel impossible!**

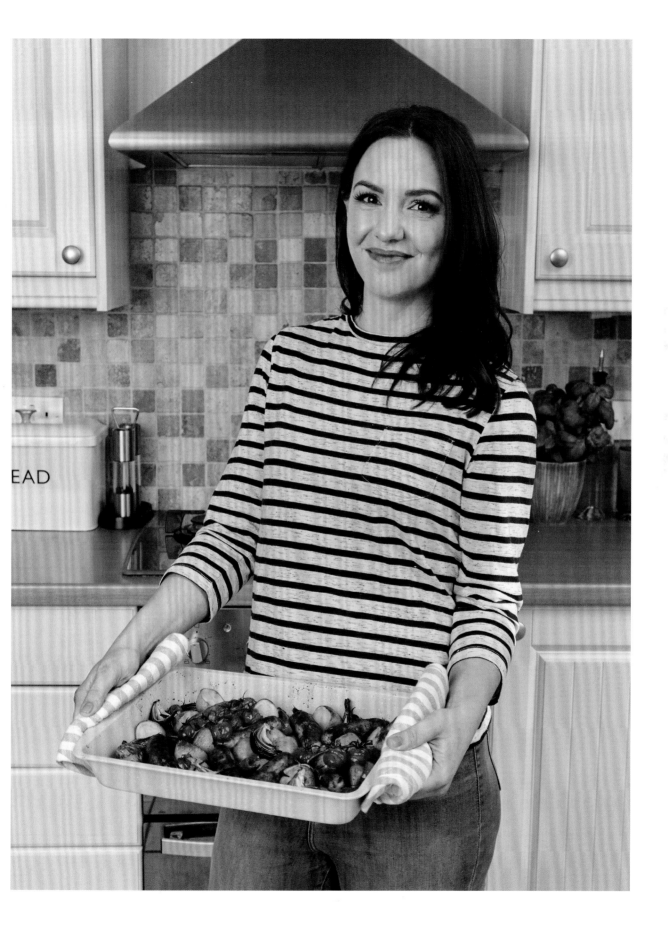

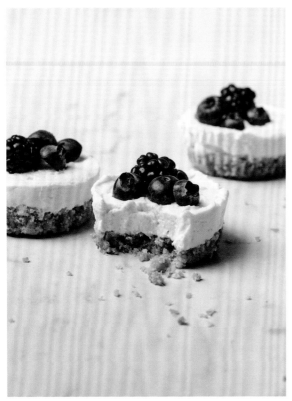
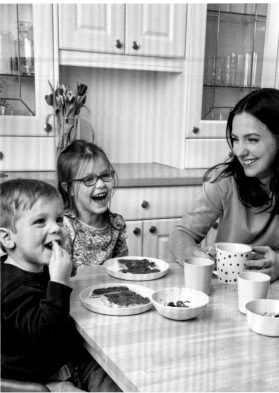
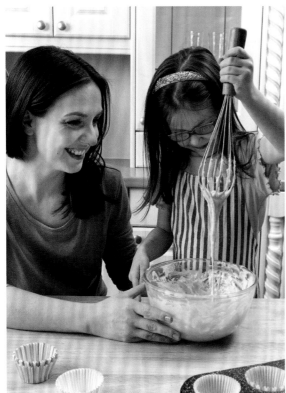
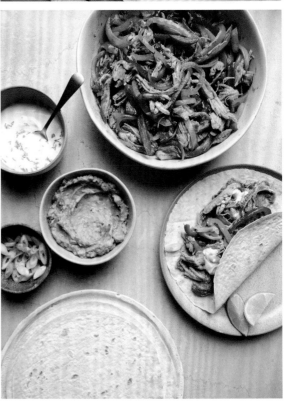

As a busy mum, one of my other priorities when developing recipes is that they are simple and fuss-free. You won't find fancy ingredients or elaborate methods – just delicious, hearty home cooking. All 65 recipes are dairy and soya free, with a handy allergen key and tips on how to adapt for weaning age.

How to use this book

As well as inspiring you with scrumptious meals that you cook for your family again and again, this book is here to empower you with information and advice and to help grow your confidence in how to navigate your allergy parent journey.

Starting with understanding what CMPA is, the different types and key symptoms to look for, we'll also explore what your allergy journey might look like from diagnosis to potential milk reintroduction. We'll cover nutrition, including milk alternatives, so you can ensure your child gets the appropriate nutrients. Next, we'll have a deep dive into weaning, with a comprehensive guide on how to introduce other allergens. In my 'allergy parents' guide to life' I'll provide practical tips for some of the key milestones you'll face, including childcare, restaurants and playdates, as well as how to tackle checking food labels. Before the recipes there's a handy guide to dairy-free alternatives, and other key ingredients I always have stocked.

Throughout the book, I'll be sharing my personal experiences, plus advice that has been reviewed by dietitian Lucy's expert eye to ensure that it's scientifically correct and evidence-based. Please be aware that the information and advice throughout this book is generalised and should never replace individualised advice given by a healthcare professional.

At the back, I'll answer the questions I get asked most often from the Instagram community. There's a detailed information table for key nutrients to include in your family's diet, and I've also signposted helpful resources for further reading, plus some of the social media pages I love to follow.

I want this book to feel like a trusted friend, and hope it provides you with inspiration and comfort. I know it can feel lonely on an allergy parent journey, but trust me, you're not alone.

Now, let's get going – you've got this!

Love, Kate x

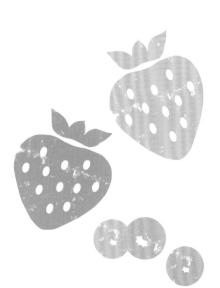

My Dairy-Free & Allergy Parent Journey

Being dairy free isn't something I ever expected to happen! I definitely used to be partial to a cheese board or box of chocolates. Then, I embarked upon a surprising rollercoaster of an allergy parent journey…

Before I became a mum, food allergies never really crossed my mind. I suffer with hay fever and also had a suspected egg allergy as a child (they used to make both my brother and I sick, but my mum didn't believe us and continued trying to hide them in meals… cheers, Mum!) However, my partner Mike has multiple allergies to food and medicine, and also had childhood asthma. I now understand that our history resulted in our kids being atopic – this means that when a parent has asthma, eczema, hay fever or food allergies their children have a higher tendency to develop allergies.

When Violet was born in 2018, we noticed pretty much straight away that something 'wasn't right'. She seemed in a lot of pain and discomfort in her tummy. As new parents, we had no idea what was 'normal'. She was exclusively breastfed and (prepare yourself for poo chat) I remember telling our health visitor at one of our post-birth home visits that she had stringy, slimy bits in her stools. This progressed quickly, until she was having eight or more loose, mucus-filled, often green, nappies a day. She was constantly pulling her legs up to her chest, screaming her lungs out and was in obvious discomfort.

She also developed dry, red eczema patches and a raised rash all over her face. I went to the GP several times, but I was told it was probably a virus, that her spots were baby acne, that 'babies cry' and was sent on my way. It was only when another friend mentioned they suspected their baby had a cow's milk allergy that I looked up the symptoms and it was like a lightbulb going on. I started a symptom diary, then when Violet was three months old, I booked to see another GP, who was wonderfully compassionate, and she suggested I eliminate all milk proteins from my diet for four weeks, then try reintroducing them.

Two weeks into the challenge Violet was so much happier, with clearer skin and more 'normal' stools. When I tried to reintroduce milk into my diet after four weeks, her pain, discomfort and tummy issues came back almost immediately, as did the rash. So I went back to the GP, who confirmed it was more than likely a milk allergy. Violet was officially diagnosed with non-IgE mediated cow's milk protein allergy (see page 18) at the allergy clinic at our local hospital a few months later. In the meantime, we were lucky enough to immediately be referred to a remote dietitian who helped to guide us through weaning and introducing other allergens.

I really struggled, however, to find dairy-free meal ideas that were suitable for her age. Having always been a foodie and passionate home cook, I decided

> # As I learned more about allergies, my passion for the subject grew, and I also started sharing advice and tips for allergy parents, plus advocating for better allergy awareness.

to start an Instagram page, documenting Violet's weaning journey and sharing the recipes I created. The Dairy Free Mum was born. I started challenging myself to create dairy-free versions of our favourite family meals and experimented with different alternatives to give the tastiest results.

As I learned more about allergies, my passion for the subject grew, and I also started sharing advice and tips for allergy parents, plus advocating for better allergy awareness. My page has grown more than I ever expected, and I'm so grateful for the amazing community that we've built together.

Meanwhile, when Violet was three, we were over the moon to be expecting again. Jude was born in 2021, and for the first few weeks we thought we'd won the parent lottery and avoided him having allergies. He was way more chilled than Violet and slept much better. He had bad reflux, but I remember I was so hopeful. Sadly, when he was seven weeks old, his skin flared up with spots and aggressive eczema, and he was constantly rubbing his face and scratching himself in his sleep. Then his gastro symptoms started showing. By this point I knew that it was more than likely a cow's milk allergy and eliminated dairy from my diet again. This time I also eliminated soya and egg, but luckily managed to reintroduce them successfully.

While I was still breastfeeding, Jude had other reactions which were treated as suspected anaphylaxis due to swollen eyes, coughing and wheezing, and we ended up at A&E twice. We've never figured out the trigger, and even now he has days where his skin flares up, he's itching uncontrollably, and we have no idea why. The second-guessing can be baffling and incredibly frustrating! At the time of writing, he's two years old and is 'stuck' on step one of the milk ladder (see page 28). Violet completed the milk ladder age three, however, and can now tolerate all dairy products, so maybe that helps to give you some hope.

On the course of this journey, we've navigated many challenges, from accidental slip-ups to frustrating comments from people who just don't get it (more on that later...) We've also, however, managed to enjoy all the milestones I once worried about so much. We've adapted, learned and grown in confidence together. Now, nothing makes me happier than us sitting all round a table together enjoying dairy-free meals I've cooked. Hopefully with the recipes in this book, you will be able to enjoy the same experience too.

part one

your dairy-free guide

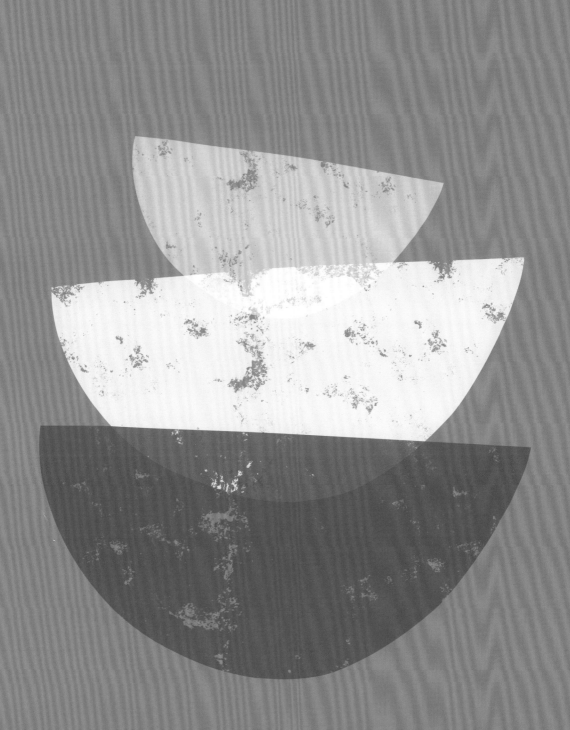

What is dairy anyway?

It's a simple question, but one that not everyone knows the answer to! Dairy products (also known as lacticinia) are food products made from, or containing, the milk of mammals e.g. cows, sheep, goats or buffaloes.

Dairy products you'll see on the shelves include butter, yoghurt, cream, cheese, custard, ghee, ice cream and, of course, milk. Many other products contain these items as an ingredient, from biscuits, cakes and sauces to ones you may not expect like stock cubes, crisps and even meat products like certain ham, sausages and chorizo. If a product contains milk, it should always be shown in bold on the label; this also includes foods containing casein, whey, buttermilk, milk powder, ghee and lactose.

Despite lots of people thinking they are, eggs are not dairy!
(eggs = chickens; milk = cows)

WHAT IS A MILK ALLERGY?

There are a few terms you might hear when talking about milk allergy – its full name is cow's milk protein allergy (CMPA or CMA). Before Violet was diagnosed, I hadn't even heard of CMPA, but over the last few years, with the help of amazing healthcare professionals like Lucy, I've learned a lot. I find it really helpful to have a basic level of understanding of the allergy itself, especially for explaining things to family and friends (who may not get what it's all about). So, in this chapter, I'll explain more about what a dairy allergy is. Some of this is quite science-y, so grab a cuppa and find yourself somewhere comfy to sit. There's also a glossary on page 216 if there are any terms you don't recognise.

Lots of people are surprised to learn that cow's milk is the most common food allergy to affect babies and young children.

Lots of people are surprised to learn that cow's milk allergy is the most common food allergy to affect babies and young children.[1] Many automatically think of peanuts when they hear the words 'food allergy' but CMPA is more prevalent, affecting somewhere between 2–7% of children under the age of one.[2]

In simple terms, milk allergy is an allergic response which is triggered by the body perceiving one, or multiple, of the proteins found in cow's milk as a threat. Basically, the immune system (incorrectly) thinks that milk proteins are dangerous, and without getting into too much medical detail, generates a response. This response is seen in the allergic symptoms experienced, which can be different for every child.

Usually, the allergy presents itself in the early weeks and months of a child's life. It could be that like my two children, symptoms show in the baby while breastfeeding by reacting to very small parts of the milk proteins that reach a mum's breast milk. More commonly, however, a reaction is seen when a baby directly ingests milk protein for the first time while weaning, in the form of infant formula or a dairy product like yoghurt.

To offer some reassurance, CMPA is outgrown in over 80% of affected children by the time they are five years old[3] and many do so between one and three years of age. Some, however, will continue to have this allergy into later childhood or adulthood.

You might be asking: why does my child have CMPA? Research is still being conducted into why certain babies are predisposed to it, but it's known that a child is more likely to develop a food allergy if the child's parents or siblings have an **atopic condition** - a food allergy, asthma, eczema or hay fever.[4] If your child themself suffers with eczema or asthma, this is also a risk factor.

IMMEDIATE VS DELAYED ALLERGY

CMPA SYMPTOMS

There are two different types of CMPA – immediate and delayed. Most children have only one type, with a small percentage experiencing both types.

Immediate (IgE mediated): symptoms display within minutes and up to two hours after ingestion. The abbreviation 'IgE' stands for *Immunoglobulin E* which is an antibody involved in sudden reactions.

Delayed (Non-IgE mediated): symptoms display between 2 and 72 hours after ingestion. This reaction isn't caused by Immunoglobulin E but usually cell reactions. This is commonly mis-labelled as intolerance (even by some healthcare professionals!) but is still an allergy, as the immune system is driving the response.

On the subject of intolerance, let's clear something up because it's something that lots of people get confused about... lactose intolerance is totally different to CMPA.

CMPA = allergy to one or more **proteins** found in cow's milk (casein and/or whey).

Lactose intolerance = a difficulty digesting lactose, the natural **sugar** found in cow's milk. It isn't an allergy because there isn't an immune response, but it can cause tummy pain and discomfort.

Lactose intolerance is actually very rare in babies, more commonly developing in adulthood. Some babies develop temporary lactose intolerance after an illness, but this will usually improve within a few weeks. CMPA symptoms wouldn't improve by switching to lactose-free products as these products contain milk proteins. So, one to be aware of, especially if someone well-meaning buys you some lactose-free cheese!

Here's a helpful summary of the most common symptoms of CMPA.

Children won't necessarily get all symptoms, but it's common to experience a range across the categories, for example a baby with delayed CMPA might get significant eczema, mucus in their stools and colic.

The vast majority won't get breathing or circulation symptoms, but if they do it's crucial to act fast as it could be anaphylaxis. Please do read page 54 for info about anaphylaxis symptoms, and what to do in an emergency.

Will my child have other allergies?

Due to the atopic link, it's more likely that your CMPA child will have other allergies, compared to a child who doesn't have an atopic condition. However, it's also possible for cow's milk to be a child's only allergy, as is the case with my children.

Soya is the most commonly linked allergy due to some similarity in the proteins in soya and cow's milk - up to 60% of CMPA babies also react to soya[5], with this largely in children with delayed CMPA. You may therefore be asked to exclude soya when undertaking a milk elimination trial, then attempt to reintroduce it. Soya allergy is also commonly outgrown, like milk allergy. Egg and peanuts are two other allergies that are (less commonly) linked to CMPA.

Immediate Symptoms (IgE mediated)	**Delayed Symptoms (Non-IgE mediated)**
Symptoms will generally appear immediately during ingestion or soon afterwards (up to 2 hours after)	*Symptoms will generally appear between 2-72 hours after ingestion*

Skin Symptoms

• Hives, nettle like rash or raised red bumps on the face and/or body (medical term: Urticaria) • Swelling, usually affecting the eyes, lips and face (medical term: Angioedema) • Itchy skin • Flushing/reddening of skin (medical term: Erythema) • Swelling usually affecting the eyes, lips and face • Sudden flare up of existing eczema	• Rash, which may come and go • Significant eczema, persisting/not improving with treatment • Itchy skin • Flushing/reddening of skin

Digestive System (Tummy and Gut) Symptoms

• Vomiting • Diarrhoea (loose/runny stools) **Note:** should vomiting or diarrhoea immediately after ingestion one or more of the above skin symptoms willl also usually be seen	• Vomiting • Reflux, bringing up mouthfuls of milk then swallowing or spitting out. Can occur with pain/discomfort, back arching, fussiness and/or irritability • Mucus and/or blood seen in stools • Constipation and/or straining to pass stools • Wind, which seems uncomfortable and excessive, may bring legs up under tummy • Diarrhoea (loose, runny stools) • Weight loss or not putting on weight

Respiratory (Breathing) Symptoms

• Difficulty in breathing that comes on suddenly • Wheeze and/or noisy breathing • Cough, that comes on suddenly and is persistent • Sneezing, runny and/or itchy nose • Hoarse voice or cry • Difficulty swallowing	Non-IgE mediated food allergies do not typically cause respiratory symptoms, if your child has symptoms such as a blocked nose, sneezing or being snuffly this will usually be caused by other factors

Appearance/Behaviour

• Floppy, pale, limp, dizzy • Sleepy or unable to stay awake	• Colic, frequent, unexplained and excessive crying • Refusal or reluctance to feed

Eczema

Both of my children suffer with eczema, so I understand how challenging it can be to deal with. For more information on triggers, treatment and things you can do to help limit your child scratching, I really recommend the National Eczema Society website (eczema.org) and booklets.

What is eczema?

Also known as dermatitis, eczema is a dry skin condition which one in five children in the UK are estimated to suffer from[6] but it can affect people of any age. It's usually a chronic condition but it can improve, or even completely resolve, as a child gets older.

What causes eczema?

Childhood eczema is more likely to develop if the child's parents or siblings suffer from eczema, asthma, allergies or hay fever (because of the atopic link). Environmental factors also play a role, including climate, temperature, pollen and dust mites, as well as individual triggers, which could include soap, sweat, food allergy, fragrance or cosmetics, clothing, animals, damp or mould, or chlorine or chemicals.

Is my child's eczema caused by a food allergy?

Food allergies like CMPA can be a trigger, but not all eczema is caused by allergies. Eczema is its own condition that needs appropriate skin management, and lots of children with eczema do not have a food allergy.

Diagnosis

If your child has symptoms of eczema - dry, itchy, cracked, inflamed or sore skin - take them to your GP who will examine them and review their history in order to make a diagnosis. For more severe cases, they may refer your child to a paediatric dermatologist. There is no cure for eczema, but treatment focuses on controlling the symptoms and preventing flare ups and possible infection.

Lucy says: *'It's exceptionally common for me to see parents who have taken one or multiple foods out of a child's diet due to their eczema. This can so often increase the risk of nutritional deficiencies, and in some cases actually increases the risk of food allergy to those foods. While food can be a trigger for eczema to persist or remain difficult to manage, even with optimised skin management, it's important to avoid lots of unnecessary food exclusions. If you suspect food to be a trigger for your child's eczema, then seek the support of an allergy specialist dietitian who can guide you through an appropriate exclusion and reintroduction plan, while ensuring your child still gets all the nutrients that they need.'*

Your allergy journey

At first, being new to the world of food allergies, I found everything pretty daunting. In our case, despite going to my GP several times concerned about Violet's symptoms, it took a long time to get to a diagnosis. I felt dismissed as an over-anxious first-time mum, and I know from your messages that this is an experience many of you share. In fact, a recent study by Allergy UK revealed that on average it can take five visits to the GP to get a diagnosis[7]. I think many in the NHS would agree that when it comes to food allergies, training and support for GPs and health visitors needs much more investment to improve awareness and management.

Once I did finally have a diagnosis, I struggled with not knowing what lay ahead. Your journey will be unique and individual to you, of course, but I've put together this example of different steps along the way to help give you an idea of what to expect.

A suspected diagnosis → referral → testing + official diagnosis → action plan + support → (possible) milk reintroduction

1. A suspected diagnosis

If you suspect CMPA, it's important to get medical advice from a GP or healthcare professional who can guide you through the appropriate steps to diagnosis.

Things to prepare for your GP appointment:

- Food diary with everything your child (and you if breastfeeding) has consumed daily in the weeks prior.
- A corresponding symptom diary with notes of any potential reactions you've been concerned about relating to skin, tummy, nappies, sleep, and anything else of interest. It can help to give symptoms a score out of ten so you can pinpoint when something has been particularly severe.
- List of formula milks previously trialled, if relevant.
- Photos and videos of any skin rashes, eczema, concerning nappies, or anything else you think is worth showing the doctor. Save these into a named album on your phone so they're easy to find on the day.

- Details of any atopic history you, your partner and your immediate family have, i.e. allergies, hay fever, eczema or asthma.
- Notes of any changes you've made so far and whether this has helped at all.
- A list of any questions you have, saved in your phone notes.

Elimination trial

In cases of suspected delayed CMPA, your GP may ask you to undertake an elimination trial. This is where your child (or you if you're breastfeeding) cuts out all milk proteins from their diet for around four weeks before reintroducing them. If symptoms improve during that time and then return when milk is reintroduced, this is usually sufficient to get a suspected diagnosis.

In cases of suspected immediate, severe CMPA or anaphylaxis, this shouldn't be done and a referral for suspected CMPA should take place without reintroduction.

Lucy says: *'If your child's symptoms have improved significantly with the exclusion of cow's milk protein, the reintroduction stage can be difficult but is such an important part of your child's diagnosis pathway. Please be reassured that a reintroduction protocol should be gradual, e.g. starting with 25g (1oz) of your child's previous milk combined with their new specialist formula, or reintroduction of cow's milk to the mother if breastfeeding at a comfortable pace.'*

2. Referral

You have a suspected CMPA diagnosis, what now? Well, your GP should hopefully refer you to an allergy clinic or local dietetic team for support. I say hopefully because unfortunately it's not always this easy, and it may be something you have to push for.

My best advice would be to trust your gut and be your child's voice. Don't be afraid to ask your GP a direct question like 'Can you please refer us to the allergy clinic?' or 'How can I get access to a dietitian?'

Be aware that it can unfortunately take a long time for your NHS referral appointment to come through. The Covid pandemic created an even bigger backlog to an already very stretched service. Some areas do offer a remote dietetic service through private companies contracted by the NHS, so it's worth asking if that's an option, and you can also ask if there are any GPs within the practice with a special interest in allergy. To manage expectations, it's very possible you could be waiting 6-12 months for an appointment, so if this is you, do make sure you've checked out the resources in the back of this book.

3. Testing and official diagnosis

Your first time at the allergy clinic may feel nerve-wracking, especially if you've been waiting a long time for the day to arrive. The purpose of this appointment is for a clinician to discuss your child's history and symptoms, in order to compile an allergy-focused clinical history and confirm a suspected diagnosis.

If your child presents with immediate symptoms, it's likely they will also perform skin prick tests to support the diagnosis of any IgE mediated allergies. They then look to create an action plan so you understand what happens next and are made aware of any further support you will receive, for example from a dietitian.

Be aware that skin prick tests won't be able to be done if your child has had antihistamines (e.g. Piriton® syrup) recently. At our hospital it was five days, but if it's not outlined in your appointment letter, call in advance to ask.

Make sure your food and symptom diary is up to date, as well as the photos and videos folder, and notes of key symptoms of concern, and what has happened since

your GP referral. Also, take a list of questions - you may only be seen in clinic once or twice a year, so don't be shy to ask lots!

On the day
- Dress your child in loose, comfy clothing that's easy to get off for a weight check, and sleeves that can roll up to easily access arms for skin prick tests.
- Leave plenty of time to park if driving (hospital parking can be a nightmare!).
- Remember to pack:
  - Your child's personal child health record (red book)
  - Appointment letter
  - Any medications your child has been prescribed
  - Your food and symptom diary, plus phone with photos and/or videos
  - Notebook and pen
  - Toys for distraction - stickers, tablet, books etc, plus dummy or comforter
  - Milk, water and snacks in case of a long wait
  - Coins or bank card for parking

Allergy tests

When it comes to food allergies, it's understandable if you're just desperate for an answer. Second guessing can be so hard on parents, who would do anything to be able to know for sure what allergies their child has, so they can keep them safe and well. It's important to understand though that, unfortunately, tests won't always give you the definitive answer you're looking for.

Appropriate allergy tests can be used for children with suspected immediate allergies, as the tests are looking for IgE antibodies and will give a 'positive' or 'negative' result.

Delayed allergies do not show on these tests, however – the only test for these allergies is a period of exclusion of the allergen with eventual reintroduction. Frustrating, I know!

Skin prick tests (SPTs)
These are the most commonly used tests for children and are a quick way for allergy teams to support diagnosis of immediate allergies. Generally they're considered reliable when interpreted alongside your child's allergy-focused history.

Remember that a negative SPT doesn't mean there's no allergy, just that there isn't an **immediate** allergy. This was the case with both my kids – negative SPTs despite very clearly having CMPA.

What to expect at a SPT:
- First, you'll agree which allergens to test for, either through samples from the hospital or you may be asked to bring more unusual allergens with you in the form of the food itself. This is called prick to prick technique.
- The nurse will draw on the forearm with a pen: + and - for positive and negative controls respectively, then an indicator for each allergen.
- A drop of histamine is added to the + symbol as a positive control, and saline (salt water solution) to the - symbol as a negative control. This is just to show that the test is working and reliable.

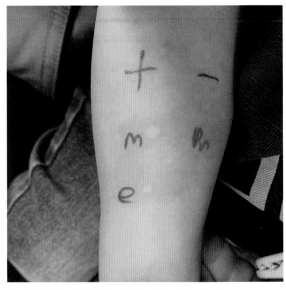

A positive SPT result indicating IgE allergies to milk and egg. Photo credit: Rachel @allergy_mummaandbubba

- The nurse will use a sharp medical tool called a lancet to 'prick' the liquid. This shouldn't hurt, but may be worrying for older children, so distraction is advised! The liquid containing the allergen will be dropped by the appropriate symbol, then the lancet will be pricked so the liquid seeps in.
- When all allergens have been pricked, you'll be asked to wait for about 15 minutes. The doctor will then assess the results of the test.
- A positive IgE result is usually confirmed if the wheal (raised hive) for an allergen is the same or larger than a positive control, or over a specific size, e.g. 3mm. Your doctor will guide you on the interpretation and significance of results. The size of the wheal does not represent the severity of allergy but instead indicates how likely it is that your child will react to that allergen. The size will be measured and noted, in order to compare to any future tests.

Blood tests

Allergy specific IgE blood tests (previously referred to as RAST tests) measure the specific amount of IgE to certain allergens. If this test is done at your allergy clinic, the results will usually take a few days or weeks to come back, which will then be interpreted and explained to you by a doctor.

My personal experience has been that clinicians seem less keen to perform blood tests on children than SPTs. While it can feel tempting as a parent to ask, 'Can't you just test for all allergies in one go?' blood tests and SPTs aren't recommended as a 'catch-all' screening test and can lead to misdiagnosis.

A note on other allergy tests

You may see testing advertised online or on social media for at home allergy, IgG, intolerance or sensitivity tests. While these can sound legitimate, please don't waste your money on them as they're not scientifically evidence-based and typically cause parents to exclude multiple foods from their own or their child's diet unnecessarily.

Lucy says: *'I always remind parents that if these home allergy tests worked for allergy diagnosis, we would absolutely use them! It can feel difficult not getting the answers you want, but please avoid resorting to these unvalidated options.'*

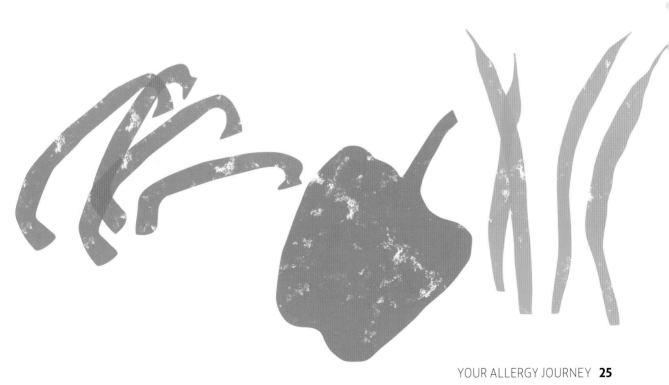

4. Action plan and support

If an immediate allergy is diagnosed, you'll be given an individualised Allergy Action Plan which outlines your medications and what situations to use them in. You'll be advised on avoiding the relevant allergens, and it'll be confirmed what ongoing support you'll receive in terms of future appointments.

Antihistamines will likely be prescribed, to be administered for any mild reactions.

Adrenaline Auto-Injectors (AAIs) are prescribed for anyone at risk of anaphylaxis, you may commonly know these as Epi-Pens. It's important, if prescribed, to always carry two with you and to make sure you're confident in how to use and store them, plus ensure that anyone else caring for your child is trained. Read more on page 54.

If a delayed allergy is confirmed, the follow-up care with the allergy clinic will depend on individual circumstances and local processes; some will see you every 6-12 months, some will discharge you to the dietitian.

For any CMPA diagnosis you should ideally be referred to a paediatric allergy dietitian. Their role is to help guide you with evidence-based and practical advice on nutrition, growth, supplements, milk, weaning, and (if delayed CMPA) tackling the milk ladder. They can also support you with practical aspects of allergy management like navigating holidays and eating out. If NHS dietetic support is not available, you can consider paying privately for appointments.

5. Milk reintroduction

As I mentioned, most children will thankfully grow out of CMPA by age five. But it isn't an overnight switch, and reintroduction needs to be handled appropriately depending on the individual circumstances of the child.

Hospital Food Challenges (for immediate allergies)

These reintroduction challenges are performed in hospitals so your child's reactions can be monitored closely by medical professionals. They will usually last around 4-6 hours where your child will gradually be given increasing amounts of the allergen, being tested every 15-20 minutes until either they react, or they tolerate the biggest portion of that step.

If they react, they'll be given appropriate medication and monitored until you're advised it's safe to go home, and you'll continue avoiding that step. However, if they tolerate the allergen, you'll be given information on how to offer it at home to maintain tolerance, and you'll be told when you will return for the next challenge, generally in a few months' time.

The challenge can only be performed if your child hasn't had any antihistamine in the days prior, so check with the hospital if you're unsure. You'll be sent details of what to take with you, including whether you need to take the food items yourself. Don't forget to pack a bag with lots of toys, books, or a tablet to keep your child entertained between doses.

IgE Allergy Parent Story

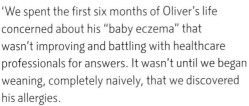

Rachel is a mum of two and runs the allergy-focused Instagram page @allergy_mummaandbubba. Her son Oliver has multiple IgE allergies.

'We spent the first six months of Oliver's life concerned about his "baby eczema" that wasn't improving and battling with healthcare professionals for answers. It wasn't until we began weaning, completely naively, that we discovered his allergies.

We had given him some baby porridge (containing cow's milk) one morning and around five minutes into eating it he began to grumble in his highchair; by the time I had taken him out and carried him into the next room, his lips and eyes were visibly swelling. Panicked, I laid him down and phoned 111 for advice, but before I could get through to anyone, he projectile vomited everywhere. I could see that hives were spreading across his body and he had begun to wheeze and gasp for breath. I now knew that I couldn't wait for 111 and instead dialled 999 who sent an ambulance to rush us to A&E, where they confirmed he'd suffered an anaphylactic reaction. From that moment on, our lives changed immeasurably.

Our first set of skin prick tests confirmed his IgE milk allergy and also uncovered IgE egg and peanut allergies. I can still vividly remember the overwhelm, the anxiety and the fear of what the future might hold.

Oliver is now five and has come such a long way since that first reaction. Progress has been slow and steady, with regular dietitian and consultant appointments, repeated testing and, eventually (when testing indicated he was ready), hospital-based food challenges. To date, he has had food challenges for baked egg, baked milk, loosely cooked egg and peanut; all of which he "passed", and he now regularly eats these foods.

He has successfully attended nursery, parties, playdates, sports clubs and has been abroad multiple times; all without serious reaction. He's happy, thriving and living his own version of a "normal" life. That's not to say it's easy; there's always an added layer of anxiety and plenty of behind-the-scenes preparation for everything he does in case of another serious reaction, but we never want his allergies to stop him experiencing what the world has to offer.'

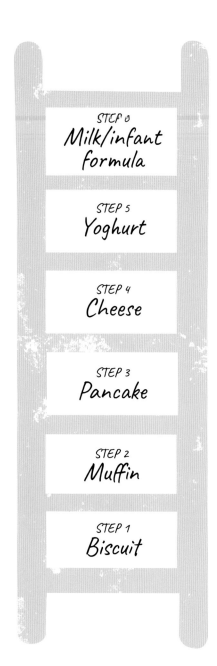

STEP 6
Milk/infant formula

STEP 5
Yoghurt

STEP 4
Cheese

STEP 3
Pancake

STEP 2
Muffin

STEP 1
Biscuit

The Milk Ladder
(for delayed CMPA)

This plan is for milk reintroduction you undertake at home, ideally guided by a dietitian.

Why a ladder?
It's called this because you introduce milk protein in increasing steps. So rather than just giving your child a pot of yoghurt and hoping for the best, you go slowly and start with a very low dose of milk protein, modifying how the protein is cooked, e.g. time or temperature, working your way up, determining what their tolerance is along the way.

When to start?
Generally around the age of 12 months or when your child has been on a milk-free diet and been symptom free for six months. Before starting you should feel confident that your child is well, their eczema is under control and they're not having any tummy symptoms so you can pinpoint any reactions more clearly.

Do you have to do it?
It can feel scary to start the milk ladder; you may worry about causing your child distress, pain, or interrupted sleep. Sometimes I'm asked 'Can't I just keep them on a milk-free diet and not risk it?' but there are lots of benefits to understanding how much, or little, your child can tolerate and then maintain that tolerance. As someone who's tackled it twice, I promise there's a definite weight off your shoulders once you get going, even if you don't get past step one first time around – at least you know!

Our milk ladder journey
Violet started the milk ladder at 11 months old (she'd been milk free for six months) with the guidance of our dietitian. She passed steps 1 and 2 straight away, then was 'stuck' on step 3 for over a year, with the usual illnesses and teething also getting in the way! She then got to step 5 but couldn't tolerate milk in its pure form for another year, before eventually completing it age three. Currently, Jude gets itchy spots and eczema flare ups from three-quarters of a biscuit (step 1), so we are waiting to try again soon.

The iMAP 6-step milk ladder

This is one of the most commonly recommended milk ladders in the UK[8] and the one we followed, but you may have been guided to follow a different ladder such as a 12-step one. As you can see opposite, the six steps are Biscuit → Muffin → Pancake → Cheese → Yoghurt → Milk/infant formula.

How much of each step you offer to begin with can differ depending on circumstances and how you're guided by your healthcare professional, based on your child's history. Personally, I've always started small – a quarter of a biscuit for example. This first amount is offered every day for an agreed number of days (commonly three days is used), to give you time to spot any delayed reactions.

If no reaction is seen, you move to a bigger quantity every day for three days and so on. Then when the step is complete, you start with a small portion of the next step.

If your child reacts, you should stop giving the food on that step of the milk ladder. However, you should continue to offer any steps that have been tolerated regularly (a few times a week) in order to maintain tolerance. So, if your child reacts at step 3, continue to give biscuits (step 1) and muffins (step 2) often. You should be guided by your dietitian when to try the 'failed' step again, but this is generally a few months after the reaction.

What if you're not sure if something is a reaction?

The number of times I've wished for a magic machine that tells you this! It can be so hard when symptoms can be similar to teething, illnesses and sometimes just developmental. The second-guessing can be really tough. The general advice would be to follow your instinct; if it seems like a reaction, then pause and try that same step/portion once symptoms are under control. If the same thing happens again, then it's more likely it was a reaction. Keeping a detailed food diary can really help here.

Try not to feel disheartened if you don't progress quickly – it might take several attempts, and you may be stuck on a step for ages. But try to keep positive and hopefully you'll get there in the end.

Step by step

The recommended approach for steps 1–3 is to follow the iMAP recipes[9] included on the following pages, so that there's an appropriate and consistent amount of milk protein per portion. The recipes have also been carefully planned to have a lower sugar content than their equivalent pre-packaged items. They are also egg and soya free, and have a wheat-free option, which is helpful should you be dealing with multiple allergies.

However, as busy parents it's understandable if it isn't always possible to make your own, so there are also shop-bought alternatives listed for the relevant steps. Always check ingredients as brands differ, may change their ingredients and some may not contain milk (it feels very weird purposefully choosing products with milk in after avoiding it for so long!). Make sure you choose products that list milk powder or milk as an ingredient, not simply 'whey'. This is because milk contains both casein and whey proteins, so if a product just contains whey, then you are not testing tolerance to casein.

STEP 1: **Biscuit**

Portion: start with either a quarter, half or whole biscuit (as recommended by your healthcare professional) and build up to three biscuits, tolerated daily for three consecutive days.

Makes 20 finger-sized biscuits

125g (4½oz) plain flour (*if using wheat-free flour, add ¼ tsp xanthan gum*)

1 tsp skimmed milk powder (found near the UHT milk in the supermarket)

50g (1¾oz) cold dairy-free butter alternative or margarine, cubed

SWEET OPTION

50g (1¾oz) grated apple, pear or mashed banana

2 drops of vanilla extract

SAVOURY OPTION

40g (1½oz) dairy-free cheese alternative, grated

10ml (2 tsp) water

1. In a bowl, mix together the flour and milk powder (*plus xanthan gum, if using*).
2. Rub in the dairy-free butter alternative or margarine.
Sweet option: Mix in the fruit and vanilla extract, adding a little more fruit if the dough seems too dry.
Savoury option: Mix in the grated cheese alternative and water. If the dough is too dry, add a splash more water.
3. Wrap the dough in clingfilm and put in the fridge for 30 minutes and preheat the oven to 180°C/350°F/Gas Mark 4.
4. On a lightly floured surface roll out the dough to 1-2cm thick and cut into 20 equal-sized finger-length strips or biscuit shapes, ensuring you use all the dough.
5. Place on a baking tray lined with baking paper and bake for 10-15 minutes until golden.
6. Cool and serve.

Shop-bought alternatives
Malted milk biscuits, Nice biscuits, digestive biscuits, shortcake biscuits, kids' biscotti.

STEP 2: **Muffin**

Portion: start with a quarter or half a muffin and build up to a whole muffin, tolerated daily for three consecutive days.

Makes 10

250g (9oz) plain flour (*if using wheat-free flour, add ½ tsp xanthan gum*)

2½ tsp baking powder

2 tbsp sugar (I use caster sugar)

pinch of salt (optional)

250ml (9fl oz) milk (whole or semi-skimmed)

50ml (2fl oz) sunflower or rapeseed (canola) oil

SWEET OPTION

110g (3¾oz) finely chopped or mashed fruit, such as apple, pear or banana

vanilla extract, to taste (optional)

SAVOURY OPTION

60g (2¼oz) dairy-free cheese alternative, grated

1. Preheat the oven to 180°C/350°F/Gas Mark 4 and line a muffin tin with 10 muffin cases.
2. In a large bowl, mix together the flour, baking powder, sugar and salt (*plus xanthan gum, if using*).
3. In a separate bowl, whisk together the milk and oil, then add to the dry mixture.
Sweet option: Add the chopped fruit and vanilla extract (if using) and fold together.
Savoury option: Add the grated cheese alternative and mix, adding a splash of water if needed.
4. Spoon the mixture equally into the 10 cases.
5. Bake for 15-20 minutes, then cool.

Shop-bought alternatives
Plain fairy cakes or muffins (with no chocolate or icing or buttercream), brioche (without chocolate), plain naan, scones.

STEP 3: **Pancake**

Portion: start with a quarter or half a pancake and build up to a whole pancake, tolerated daily for three consecutive days.

Makes 6

125g (4½oz) plain flour (wheat or wheat free)

2½ tsp baking powder

¼ tsp salt (optional)

2 tbsp sunflower or rapeseed (canola) oil, plus extra for frying

250ml (9fl oz) milk (whole or semi-skimmed)

50ml (2fl oz) water

1. Add all the ingredients to a large bowl and mix well.
2. Heat a frying pan on a medium heat with a little oil.
3. Add a ladle of the mixture into the pan and fry on both sides until cooked through (the consistency is like crêpes rather than fluffy pancakes).

If your child won't eat pancakes, there is an option of using cooked potato, which is detailed in the iMAP guideline recipes. This option would be considered more allergenic compared to pancakes.

Shop-bought alternatives
Scotch pancakes (no chocolate), frozen Yorkshire puddings, sweet waffles or croissants.

STEP 4: **Cheese**

Portion: building up to 15g (½oz) hard cheese (e.g. Cheddar or Edam) tolerated daily for three consecutive days.

Once this is tolerated, you can introduce baked cheese in dishes such as lasagne, pizza etc. If your child doesn't like the taste, try sprinkling some onto their favourite meal and mixing in.

STEP 5: **Yoghurt**

Portion: building up to 125ml (4fl oz) yoghurt tolerated daily for three consecutive days.

Choose a plain or Greek-style yoghurt and sweeten with fruit if required. After yoghurt, you should be able to try butter, chocolate and soft cheese.

STEP 6: **Milk/Infant Formula**

Portion: start with 100ml (3½fl oz) pasteurised milk/infant formula and mix this with current milk replacement. Build up to 200ml (7fl oz). If this is tolerated, you can switch all current milk replacements (bottle and in breakfast cereals) to pasteurised milk or suitable infant formula.

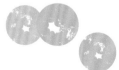

Nutrition

Worrying about whether you or your child are getting enough nutrients on a dairy-free diet is completely understandable. It's a big deal to cut out a major food group, and it shouldn't be taken lightly. However, I promise that with some consideration it's possible to get everything you need when following a balanced, nutritious milk-free diet.

When I first got Violet's diagnosis, I had these worries, so I made it my mission to become a bit of a dairy-free 'nutrition nerd', basically so I could feel confident I was feeding her the right foods to support growth and development. If you're a CMPA parent, you'll ideally be guided with individualised nutrition advice from a paediatric dietitian, but if you're on the waiting list it's good to know the basics before then.

In this chapter we'll go through the important nutrients for when you're dairy free and tips for achieving a healthy balanced diet.

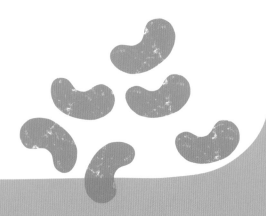

KEY NUTRIENTS WHEN DAIRY FREE

Taking care to include key nutrients is crucial to achieving a healthy diet when dairy free. Cow's milk is naturally nutrient-rich, so avoiding it means finding these elsewhere in the diet.

In the back of the book you'll find a chart with the different nutrients and why they're important, guideline daily requirements and good dairy-free sources. The key ones to be conscious of are:

Macronutrients

We need these nutrients in large amounts to provide us with energy, and they should usually form the biggest part of meals we serve.

Starchy carbohydrates – these give the body important vitamins and fibre. Found in potatoes, pasta, rice and grains, bread and oats.

Protein – essential for muscle growth and repair. Found in eggs, fish, meat, legumes (beans, lentils and chickpeas), nuts and seeds, quinoa and soya products like tofu and soya yoghurt or milk.

Fats – provide the body with essential fatty acids (omega-3 and omega-6). Some fat in the diet is important, but you should try to avoid too much saturated fat, which is found in biscuits, cakes etc. Healthy fat sources include oily fish, seeds, nuts, vegetable oils, avocado and olives.

Micronutrients

These nutrients are needed by the body in very small amounts but are essential for good health.

Calcium – if you're dairy free you may already be worrying about calcium intake. Needed for maintaining strong bones and teeth, it's a crucial one. Ensure your plant-based alternatives for milk, cheese and yoghurts are calcium-fortified and look for fortified breads and cereals. Also found in canned fish, oranges, white beans, chia seeds and green leafy vegetables like broccoli, spring greens and bok choy.

Iodine – one I'd never heard of before being dairy free but is really important for production of thyroid hormones and supporting the development of baby's brain during pregnancy, infancy and early childhood. Good sources include white fish and shellfish, eggs, and iodine-fortified milk and yoghurt alternatives.

Iron – needed for making red blood cells and muscle development during growth. Babies are born with iron stores which last until they're around six months old before declining, so iron is an important nutrient to include in the diet regularly. Iron-rich sources include red meat, fish, poultry, eggs and offal. Plant-based iron sources like legumes, dark green vegetables, nuts and seeds are absorbed less easily, but eating a vitamin C source with the meal can help with the absorption of iron.

Vitamin A (retinol) – helps the immune system work properly, keeps skin healthy and aids vision in dim light. Found in eggs, oily fish and fortified products like margarine. You can also get vitamin A by including good sources of beta-carotene in your diet as the body can convert this into retinol; try yellow, red and green (leafy) vegetables like spinach, carrots, sweet potatoes and red peppers plus yellow fruit like mango, papaya and apricots.

B Vitamins - essential for helping to release energy from food and keeping the skin, eyes and nervous system healthy. Look for fortified plant-based milk alternatives; they are also found in eggs, fortified breakfast cereals, mushrooms, meat, fish and eggs.

Vitamin C - helps to protect cells and keep them healthy, supporting the immune system, and maintains healthy skin, bones and blood vessels. Include good sources in the diet regularly, including citrus fruits, tomatoes, peppers, broccoli, strawberries and potatoes.

Vitamin D - aids the absorption of calcium and phosphate into the body to maintain strong bones, muscles and teeth. In the spring and summer we get most of our vitamin D from sunlight, but as babies and young children shouldn't be exposed to the sun, daily vitamin D supplements are recommended (see page 36). It's also important to include food sources such as fortified products, eggs, red meat, oily fish and mushrooms.

Zinc - important for immune function, growth and development. Found in meat, shellfish, legumes, nuts and seeds.

Meeting their nutritional needs

Please don't feel you need to calculate individual nutrient amounts for every meal - that's a sure-fire way to stress yourself out. A much easier, and more achievable, goal is to aim to offer a healthy balance *across the day*, or even *over the course of a week*.

Some meals will be naturally higher in some nutrients than others, and days will vary for different reasons. Sometimes even if you plan everything to perfection, your child will flat out refuse certain foods, or it'll end up on the floor! So thinking of it as a bigger picture gives you more flexibility (and sanity…).

Meeting the daily requirements of individual nutrients might be easier than you think. Let's take calcium and iodine requirements for a 1-2 year old, for example:

Calcium - daily requirement of 350mg could be met by consuming:
- 200ml (7fl oz) plant-based milk alternative that is fortified with 120mg calcium per 100ml (240mg) PLUS
- 30g (1oz) serving of Cheerios® multigrain cereal (161mg) OR
- 1 orange (approx. 70mg) AND 1 slice of bread (approx. 49mg)

Iodine - daily requirement of 70mcg could be met by consuming:
- 200ml (7fl oz) plant-based milk alternative that is fortified with 22mcg per 100ml (44mcg) PLUS
- 1 fish finger (approx. 30mcg) OR
- 1 egg (approx. 26mcg)

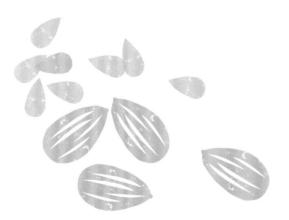

A healthy balanced diet

Once your child gets to the age of one, these recommendations[10] to achieve a healthy, balanced diet for children up to the age of five are helpful as a general guide:

- 5 portions of starchy carbohydrates per day
- 5 portions of fruit and veg per day
- 3 servings of calcium-rich food per day
- 2 portions of iodine-rich food per day
- 2 servings of protein and iron-rich food per day
- Plenty of water, at mealtimes and in between
- Maximum 2 servings of foods high in saturated fat and sugar (e.g. cakes, biscuits) per week
- No added salt in cooking and limited salty snacks
  - <12 months - less than 1g salt per day
  - 1-3 years - less than 2g salt per day
  - 4-6 years - less than 3g salt per day

How I approach it

- I always meal plan on a weekly basis. The recipes in this book have been built with key nutrients in mind and those that are particularly high in calcium, iodine, iron and/or protein are mentioned in the recipe notes.

- Choosing fortified plant-based milk, yoghurt and cheese alternatives helps (see page 41 for some tips on these) and I look for products like cereal and bread with extra vitamins added.

- I often put together a 'picky plate' for lunch or tea (basically a selection of random bits from the fridge or cupboards... Violet loves them!) as this can be a great way of offering different nutrient-rich foods in a fun way for kids. An example could be:
  - canned tuna or mashed beans mixed with fortified yoghurt (protein, iron, iodine)
  - toast, pitta bread or tortilla wrap (energy, calcium)
  - berries or oranges (vitamin C, to help aid iron absorption)
  - avocado or 100% nut butter (healthy fats)

- While fresh, homemade food is undoubtedly brilliant, I also appreciate the reality of parenthood. Yes, despite writing a cookbook, I do serve my kids freezer dinners of fish fingers, potato smiles and peas or beans. These meals do actually offer plenty of nutritional value (iodine, energy, protein, fat, calcium, vitamin C), so don't beat yourself up for offering them, just be aware of the saturated fat and salt levels of processed foods and try to also offer home-cooked meals where possible.

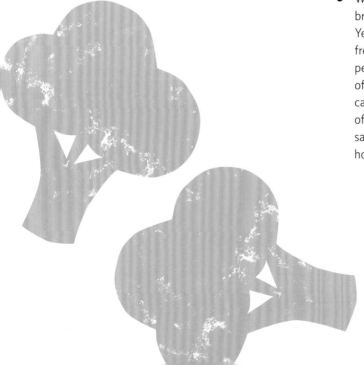

Supplements when dairy free

Here's what you should be offering in terms of vitamin supplements. If you're not already, don't stress - just buy some now and include them in your daily routine.

Babies (0–6 months) - if breastfed or if formula fed/combination fed but consuming less than 500ml (18fl oz) formula per day you should give a daily vitamin D drop containing 8.5-10mcg.

6 months–5 years - if breastfed or if formula fed but consuming less than 500ml (18fl oz) formula per day, you should give a daily vitamin drop of vitamins A, C and D.

Adults - 10mcg vitamin D per day during autumn and winter (or all year round if higher risk e.g. people who are frail or housebound, are in an institution such as a care home, or usually wear clothes that cover most of their skin when outdoors).[11]

WHEN BREASTFEEDING

Your nutritional needs jump massively when breastfeeding, and avoiding dairy can make this more challenging. The key requirements to be aware of on top of vitamin D are:

Calcium: 1,250mg per day (nearly double the normal daily requirement!)
Iodine: 200mcg per day[12]

Make sure you're taking a multivitamin or individual supplements to meet these needs, alongside including natural sources in your diet. Many multivitamins are available now specifically for breastfeeding mums, which include good levels of these, plus lots of other vitamins and minerals. Always check vitamin supplements for allergens, as some brands contain peanut oil, soya or others.

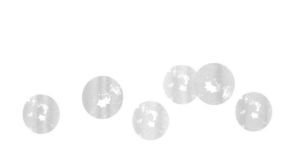

MILK

This can feel like such a confusing topic when dairy free and is one of the areas I get asked about the most. My inbox is constantly buzzing with questions like 'Should I give up breastfeeding?', 'How can I get my baby to accept prescription formula?', 'Which plant-based milk alternative is best for my toddler?', 'What age can they have it from?' So let's dive in and get your questions answered!

Breastfeeding on a dairy-free diet

Breast milk has a multitude of benefits for baby and mum, including helping to lower the risk of baby getting infections, sudden infant death syndrome (SIDS) and mum getting certain cancers. Current World Health Organization guidance recommends exclusive breastfeeding to six months of age, and continued breastfeeding until your baby is two years old.[13]

It's totally possible to breastfeed while avoiding dairy, but it's important to be aware of your own nutritional needs at this time, so take note of the advice on page 36.

CMPA can occur in breastfed babies, but research suggests it's much less common (0.5–1%) than in formula-fed babies (2–7.5%).[14] If your baby reacts through your breastmilk, you'll need to cut out all milk proteins from your diet, first for the elimination trial (see page 22), then if CMPA is confirmed for the duration of breastfeeding, until the milk ladder is underway. It's possible you may also need to avoid soya for the elimination trial, as cross-reaction between these two allergens can be more common.

Your baby may react to cow's milk directly (through eating) but not through your breastmilk. If this is the case, then you don't need to adjust your diet, just your child's.

If your baby is diagnosed with CMPA, you can absolutely continue to breastfeed, and have a positive feeding journey. You shouldn't feel pressured to stop breastfeeding if you don't want to. There are many wonderful reasons to breastfeed, and the experience can be incredibly rewarding. I'm not going to sit here and say it will be easy though. If you've previously eaten dairy regularly, it can feel like a major change to suddenly cut it out completely. Don't underestimate that it'll have an impact on you, mentally as well as physically. As a large food group it's important to consider the energy contribution too - breastfeeding increases the energy demands of mum each day, so many avoiding dairy may be at risk of not meeting their daily energy requirements.

If you're struggling

- Don't give up breastfeeding on a bad day. Write down how you're feeling and come back to it the next day.

- Chat to your health visitor and share any concerns you have and consider additional professional support from an IBCLC (International Board Certified Lactation Consultant) if needed.

- Try to find others who are on the same journey - consider joining a local breastfeeding support group or search for 'Breastfeeding with CMPA' groups online.

- Be kind to yourself - your feeding journey is personal to you, and it's your opinion that matters most. If you don't want to continue breastfeeding, that's OK too.

Specialist formula

If you choose to formula feed/combination feed and your baby is dairy free, it's frustratingly not as simple as popping to the local supermarket to pick up a different tub of milk.

Soya formula (e.g. SMA® Wysoy) is available to buy, which is suitable if you are dairy free for lifestyle reasons, like following a vegan diet, but is currently not recommended for milk allergy babies under the age of six months due to the phytoestrogen content (see Q&A, page 208) and increased risk of soya sensitivity.

For CMPA babies, it's also not advised to use goat's milk formula as the proteins of goat's milk are similar to cow's milk so typically children cross-react.

There are two types of hypoallergenic (specialist) formula for CMPA babies available, either of these would need to be prescribed by your GP:

EXTENSIVELY HYDROLYSED FORMULA (EHF)

Examples include: Nutramigen LGG®, Similac® Alimentum, Aptamil® Pepti, SMA® Althéra

These formulas still contain cow's milk but the proteins which cause the reaction are broken down (hydrolysed) into smaller pieces, making it much less likely a child will react to them.

EHFs are tolerated by around 90% of CMPA babies[15] and will usually be prescribed first, before making any decision to use an amino acid formula, unless otherwise directed by a healthcare professional.

AMINO ACID FORMULA (AAF)

Examples include: Neocate®, SMA Alfamino®, Nutramigen Puramino®, Similac® Elecare

These formulas don't contain any intact cow's milk proteins, instead being made from amino acids. They are typically required by around 10% of babies who react to EHF or may be a first port of call for babies who have experienced more severe symptoms like anaphylaxis.

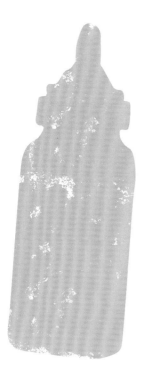

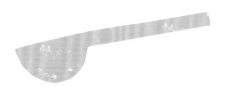

- Always check the specific preparation instructions, as these can vary and are different from cow's milk formula. For example, you may need to use water that has been boiled then cooled to room temperature.

- Getting your baby to accept it can have its challenges as it tastes pretty vile! If you're really struggling here are some things you can try:
  - Mix with your breastmilk or current formula and slowly adjust the amount of the specialist formula until they accept. For example, mix 4 parts current milk to 1 part specialist formula, then when they are happy with this, move to 3 parts current milk to 2 parts specialist formula and so on. The only exception to this would be when a baby has a suspected or confirmed immediate allergy.
  - Dip the bottle teat in their current milk to help encourage acceptance.
  - Experiment with feeding positions or different people offering feeds.
  - Try to stay calm and don't force feed if they're really upset. Take a break and try again later to avoid creating negative associations.
  - As a last resort, and if discussed with a healthcare professional, add a tiny amount of (alcohol-free) vanilla extract or (dairy-free) strawberry flavour milkshake liquid or powder into the bottle to help disguise the flavour, then wean down. This isn't ideal, as they contain sugar, but is the only way Jude accepted it at first! I started with ⅛ teaspoon of strawberry milkshake powder per bottle, then weaned the amount down over the space of two weeks until he happily accepted it without.

- Specialist formulas can turn baby's stools a dark green colour and also change the frequency and consistency, which is normal, but may give you a fright at first!

- If your baby suffers with reflux, you may be advised to use a thickener with specialist formula. Always discuss suitable options with your healthcare professional as some contain allergens.

- It can take time for your baby to adjust when changing to a new formula, so it's usually recommended to wait a few weeks before discussing with a healthcare professional whether it's suitable or not.

- Check with your GP surgery the easiest way of ordering repeat prescriptions and speak to your pharmacy about stock levels (they often have to order it in, which can take a few days). If you ever find yourself in a situation where you don't have the formula you need, call 111 for advice.

- Amino acid formulas in particular are very expensive to produce and incur a high cost for the NHS. A lot of you have shared stories with me that you have struggled to get prescribed enough cans or been made to feel guilty when collecting prescriptions. I personally experienced this, and as a parent it made me so upset – if this is what's required for your child's health, you should never be made to feel guilty for needing it, in the same way as any other medicine. So if you ever encounter this, don't be afraid to be direct if you need to, and advocate for your child. A clear letter from your dietitian can also help in these cases too.

" My Feeding Story

I've had two completely different feeding journeys with my children. Violet was exclusively breastfed, and I was lucky that I had a really positive breastfeeding experience. I loved the closeness and bond it helped to create, and the feeling that I could soothe and comfort her with my milk. Plus the fact that I didn't have to wash bottles and remember to pack them when I went out was a big bonus! When she was diagnosed with CMPA, it was tough cutting out all dairy, but I continued to enjoy breastfeeding. I did try offering an expressed bottle of breastmilk at various points, but she never accepted it and instead moved on to a cup of fortified oat milk when she was a year old.

With Jude, my plan was to do the same, but his reactions made breastfeeding incredibly stressful for me. Whenever he had a flare up, even after I'd cut out dairy, I drove myself crazy wondering what I'd eaten to cause it (when it probably wasn't even food related). At one point I'd cut out dairy, soya, eggs and nuts from my diet. I was miserable, had very little energy and had lost a lot of weight.

When Jude was hospitalised at four months old because of a severe reaction, he was weighed, and we realised he was dropping centiles on his growth chart. A kind consultant chatted to me for a while, and when she asked how I was feeling about breastfeeding I ended up bursting into tears. I admitted it wasn't making me happy and was worried it wasn't the healthiest option for him, or me, as things stood.

We ended up making the decision to move him to extensively hydrolysed formula at the hospital. After a couple of weeks his CMPA rash and tummy issues had returned, however, and he was then moved to an amino acid formula which settled all his symptoms. Moving to formula was absolutely the right choice for us, I was a lot happier once we'd switched over and enjoyed the freedom of other people being able to feed him too.

Hopefully, what my story tells you is that there isn't one 'right' way to feed. It's possible you may be reading this feeling the dreaded mum guilt either way:

'I'm breastfeeding but I feel guilty that my child is having reactions through my milk.'

'I'm formula feeding but I feel guilty that I "should" be breastfeeding.'

Well, I'm here having fed both ways to say that the correct decision is **your** decision.

"

Plant-based milk alternatives
Let's call them PBMAs for the sake of my word count!

There's such a broad range of PBMAs available now, with new ones launching every year and many brands now offering 'growing up' versions specifically for children.

The first thing to note is that PBMAs should not be offered as a main drink until your baby is at least **one year old** - they should continue with breastmilk or formula milk until then. You can, however, use PBMA in cooking, on cereal and porridge from six months of age. When your baby reaches one, your GP may stop your prescription for specialist formula, and ask you to switch to a PBMA.

CHOOSING A PBMA

- Types of milk generally advised for children over the age of one are based on soya or pea (due to the higher protein content in these) or oat. Unless your baby is allergic to all of these, in which case consult your dietitian.
  - Avoid rice milk for under-fives due to arsenic content.
  - Coconut and nut-based milks (e.g. almond) are generally too low in calories and protein.
  - Avoid **organic** PBMAs as they aren't fortified with important vitamins and minerals.
- Opt for unsweetened versions where possible.
- Look for ones with higher calorie, protein and fat levels - aim for one that per 100ml (3½fl oz) has 50 or more calories, 1g protein and 3g fat. If your child's PBMA is a lower protein option, e.g. oat, then aim to include protein-rich sources in their diet.
- Ensure the PBMA is fortified with:
  - calcium (aim for 120mg or more per 100ml/3½fl oz)
  - iodine (aim for 22mcg or more per 100ml/3½fl oz)
  - vitamins D and B12
- You may find your baby, or you, prefers the taste of some milks to others, and this is important too! I've personally always preferred barista-style oat milk in my coffee, and soya milk in my tea, whereas even though Jude can tolerate soya, he doesn't seem to like the taste, so has oat milk as his main drink.

SOME MORE HANDY TIPS

- PBMAs can be eye-wateringly expensive, especially when you're going through a lot of cartons, so shop around and take advantage of supermarket offers. You can also find some available for bulk delivery or monthly subscription.
- Consider buying two types - one that ticks the boxes above for your child's main drink, and a cheaper version for cooking or cereal (check it's still fortified with calcium and iodine though). Don't instantly dismiss the supermarket brands as many are now coming close to the branded ones in terms of nutrition and are much cheaper.
- Don't forget to shake the carton every time you use it, as some nutrients like calcium settle in a sediment that falls to the bottom of the carton.

> **Lucy says**: *'As of yet there isn't one particular PBMA that hits the nutritional mark across all fronts, so you may need to compromise somewhere and decide which one works best for you, taking into consideration the above and also personal factors such as budget. If a nutrient is lower or missing, dietetic support should help you identify where else this can be found.'*

Weaning & introducing allergens

Introducing your baby to solid food is an important milestone as a parent, and weaning can be a really fun and rewarding experience (not to mention messy…!)

Add in your child having a food allergy, however, and it can cause a lot of worry and stress. For me, knowing my kids had allergies before our weaning journey made me quite anxious about the process, especially about introducing other allergens.

This chapter aims to provide you with key information and advice to help support your journey. First, we'll go through the basics including when to start weaning, the different approaches and which foods to avoid. You'll then find my top weaning tips and how to approach the first few weeks before your baby is ready to eat the meals in this book. Finally, there's important guidance on the most common allergens and how to introduce them, the different types of reaction you might encounter and what to do if that happens.

INTRODUCTION TO WEANING
AKA COMPLEMENTARY FEEDING/STARTING SOLIDS

In the UK, the current guidance is to start weaning around six months of age, but not before 17 weeks. Solid foods should be offered alongside breastfeeding and/or formula milk.

As well as being around six months of age, your baby should be showing all the developmental signs that they're ready for food. Namely being able to:

- Stay in a sitting position holding their head steadily, so they can swallow food and eat safely.
- Coordinate their eyes, hands and mouth, so for example look at food, pick it up and put it in their mouth. This is so they can eat independently, and self-feeding can be supported from the start of weaning.
- Swallow food, rather than spit it out. You may have heard of the 'tongue thrust reflex' which babies have in the first few months of life, and usually lose around 4-6 months old. Prior to weaning, this should have diminished. If, when you put a spoon to their lips, they automatically push it out with their tongue, they still have the reflex and aren't developmentally ready yet.

There are two main methods of weaning:
Purées (aka spoon feeding) – where food is blended and offered to baby on a spoon. To begin with, baby is offered smooth purées and then progresses through textures, getting lumpier over time.
Baby-led – where you offer suitable finger foods for your baby to feed themselves from the start of weaning (often just adapting the family meal).

Many choose to do a mix of both methods, offering both finger food and purées, so don't feel you have to pick one method and stick to it religiously. Flexibility is key, and you'll find all babies are completely different in terms of the weaning style they best respond to.

Early weaning

If your baby is considered higher risk for food allergies you **may** be advised to start weaning earlier, from four months old, with the close support of a healthcare professional.

Higher risk would be if they have:
- An existing allergy (e.g. if they have already been diagnosed with CMPA) and/or
- Eczema (particularly if their eczema is severe, e.g. needs regular steroid treatment)

Research indicates that high-risk babies may benefit from early introduction to eggs and peanuts specifically to help prevent these food allergies developing.[16] Studies are ongoing into the potential benefits of introducing other allergens earlier than six months.

The decision to wean prior to six months of age should always be guided by a dietitian or allergist based on your individual circumstances. If you do wean early, it's still important that your baby is showing the developmental readiness signs, and that you get additional support where needed on things like feeding methods and seating positions. Typically it's recommended to follow a purée approach before six months old, rather than baby-led weaning.

What to avoid

If your child has already been diagnosed with CMPA, it's important to totally avoid giving them any milk proteins during weaning (see guidance on milk reintroduction on page 26).

There are several other foods to avoid:

Salt - avoid adding to baby's meals completely, including ingredients like stock cubes, and be aware of their salt intake from packaged foods like bread, cereals and dairy alternatives.

Sugar - it can cause tooth decay and displace intake of other key nutrients during weaning and the early years.

Honey - this must be completely avoided before your baby is 12 months old, as it can occasionally contain bacteria that can produce toxins in a baby's intestines, leading to a very serious illness called botulism.

Whole nuts and certain nut butters - these should be avoided before five years of age due to being a choking hazard. Chunky or crunchy nut butters should be avoided, and any that are thicker smooth varieties should always be mixed with a wet food and not offered undiluted directly from a spoon.

Raw eggs - only British Lion stamped eggs are safe to serve lightly cooked, or raw in something like mayonnaise. If you can't tell if they're British Lion stamped, ensure the egg is cooked through - this is also the case for duck, goose or quail eggs.

Rice milk alternative - under the age of five, children shouldn't drink rice-based drinks due to high levels of naturally occurring arsenic.

Choking hazards - common ones include popcorn, marshmallows, jelly cubes, hot dogs, round hard sweets and lollipops, raw hard fruits and veg such as apple and carrot (must be cooked), whole round fruit such as grapes, blueberries and cherry tomatoes (must be cut).

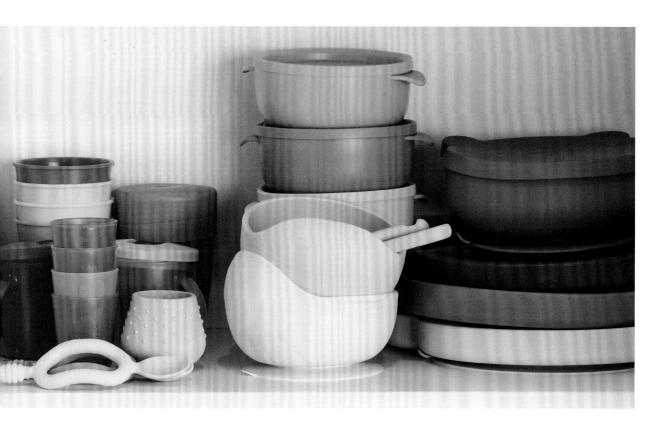

Getting kitted out

There's no need for lots of expensive equipment, but you'll want to make sure you have the basics. The key items I'd recommend are:

- A highchair with a supportive back, safety straps and, if possible, a footrest (someone once told me that a baby in a highchair without a footrest was like an adult trying to eat perched on a bar stool!)
- Washable bibs - we always used the machine washable, long-sleeved apron-style ones, which were brilliant.
- Wash cloths for wiping baby - reusable ones work really well and using just water is kindest for baby's skin.
- Hand blender or food processor if you're planning to offer purées.
- Bowls and plates - those with a suction base are handy to avoid spills.

- Spoons - ones designed for self-feeding are great, alongside more traditional soft baby purée spoons.
- Water cup - an open cup or sippy cup is best. Avoid a valved cup that encourages sucking, as the aim is to teach your baby a new drinking skill.
- Waterproof splash mat - not essential but saves a lot of mess.
- Lidded storage pots - handy for storing foods in the fridge and freezer, and for taking out and about.

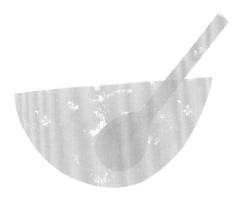

MY TOP 5 WEANING TIPS

1. Learn the difference between gagging and choking

Gagging. This is usually loud, with your baby coughing and/or spluttering and perhaps turning red in the face. It can be tough to witness, but this is actually a normal part of the weaning process as your child gets used to eating, and is a protective reflex. As your baby grows, and gains more experience with foods and textures, their gag reflex will move further back in their mouth, so they will gag less. In this event you should let your baby work the food towards the front of their mouth themselves and don't be tempted to put your fingers in their mouth as this can actually increase the risk of choking.

Choking. This is when food has blocked, or partially blocked, the airway. Choking is quiet, often silent in fact, and baby's face will turn pale or blue. Choking is an emergency, and you will need to help dislodge the food – supporting baby leaning forwards across your lap, delivering back blows. If ineffective, you should follow the baby CPR procedure and seek emergency medical attention.

I found videos and information from *Keep a Beat*[17] particularly useful, including how to take steps to avoid choking, and followed their mantra:

Loud and red – let them go ahead
Quiet and blue – they need help from you

I'd advise taking a first aid course or watching videos of what to do in the event of choking, and how to perform CPR. Being knowledgeable about what to do in an emergency will give you much more confidence.

2. Keep a food diary

Detailing which foods you have introduced on which days is a really helpful tool to be able to track progress, and also to look back at, should there be any suspected allergic reactions. There's no need to wait three days between each new food unless it's a common allergen. You may see a lot of advice online (particularly on allergy/ CMPA forums) that you should wait three days between introducing any single food. Unless otherwise advised by a healthcare professional, this isn't generally needed, and this rule is only for introducing allergens. If you only introduce one new food every three days this can create a very slow approach and impact the exposure and experience your child is getting to new foods. Variety is key when weaning, so the aim is to build up to offering lots of different tastes and textures.

3. Ensure safe food preparation

When dealing with allergies, it's important to be extra cautious when preparing food to ensure that you limit the risk of cross-contamination of the allergens you're avoiding. Always sanitise work surfaces before and after use, and anyone involved in preparing food must wash their hands thoroughly. Equipment should always be washed well between uses, and you might want to consider getting separate crockery and cutlery that only your baby uses (different colours can be helpful here).

4. Model

Your baby will learn a huge amount just by watching you eat, so always try to sit with them and have your own plate of what they are having. Try to make mealtimes relaxed and enjoyable, as your baby will pick up on your anxiety or stress. I know this isn't easy, when dealing with allergies in particular, but I used to find a fun playlist of songs helped and tried to keep my expression positive and cheerful. As well as making sure your baby is developmentally ready, consider the time you offer meals. The ideal is that they're not tired and hungry, and you have enough of a window to not have to rush the meal.

5. Try not to compare

Each baby is unique; some will take to weaning very quickly whereas others will take a lot more time. Be led by your baby's appetite and development rather than stressing too much about portion sizes or what they 'should' be eating. If you're really concerned about your child's food intake, or if they have faltering growth, always consult a healthcare professional.

The first weeks of weaning

When starting out, the aim is to introduce food in a way that allows baby to explore and learn new skills. They may not swallow anything at first, and that's OK! Milk will still be their primary source of nutrition at this point.

Many experts advise starting with bitter vegetables, to increase the likelihood of your child consuming vegetables when they're older, but it's your choice.

How I approached it

Both Violet and Jude started weaning a week or so before they turned six months, as they were showing all the signs that they were ready. With Violet, I followed baby-led weaning, using the bitter veg first approach and she took to it really well. In fact if I tried to offer anything on a spoon, she'd grab it and try to self-feed... Little Miss Independent from the beginning!

With Jude I was more relaxed about the approach (and had a lot less time to think about/prepare his food) and did a mix of finger food and purées, some homemade and some pouches. He seemed to enjoy both ways, and I found the combination easier to manage.

It is worth noting that although both my kids took to weaning well, I also had moments of panicking that they were choking (they weren't) and worrying they weren't eating when ill or teething. So it's totally normal to worry a bit!

I started with one 'meal' a day around lunchtime for the first month or so, then introduced a second meal in the morning. For the first two weeks I offered individual tastes, then built up to combinations of flavours and introducing allergens. After that point, I personally would have offered them the meals in this book, adapted where required according to the notes.

HOW TO PREPARE FOOD

To make purées, steam, boil or roast the ingredients until soft, then add to a blender with the milk they usually drink or water (enough to cover the food) and blend. Start out with the vegetables being smooth then aim to progress on to lumpier textures over the next few weeks.

Any finger food offered should be soft enough to squish between finger and thumb. Foods should be cut long and wide, in the general size and shape of your finger, for baby to be able to grasp in their fist and have the ends of the strip poking out each side.

Water can be offered alongside meals from six months old (tap water from six months or cooled boiled water prior to this). Don't worry if they don't drink much – they will be getting all their hydration from breast milk or formula still – but it's great practice for them to start learning to drink from a cup.

When should you move to more meals per day?
Every baby is different, so try not to compare too much and be led by them. You'll soon notice when they seem ready for more solids in the form of a second, and eventually third meal. Generally, most babies progress to two meals a day around 4–6 weeks into weaning, and three meals a day somewhere between 7–9 months of age.

> "
>
> **Lucy says:** *'There isn't one right way to start weaning, and I often remind parents that weaning is a process of learning to eat. It can be easy to think babies will just "get it" but in fact, eating is probably one of the most complex skills your baby will learn.'*
>
> "

FIRST FOOD IDEAS

Weeks 1 and 2: individual tastes

- Courgette (purée or steamed fingers)
- Broccoli (purée or steamed florets)
- Cauliflower (purée or steamed florets)
- Green beans (purée or steamed)
- Avocado (purée/finger-sized strips)
- Potato (mashed mixed with baby's usual milk or boiled finger-sized strips)
- Carrot (purée or steamed fingers)

- Aubergine (purée or roasted fingers)
- Sweet potato (purée or roasted fingers)
- Spinach purée
- Porridge made with baby's usual milk
- Butternut squash (purée or roasted fingers)
- Mashed banana or banana fingers
- Pear (purée or steamed fingers)

Weeks 3 and 4: combining tastes

After individual tastes, you're then ready to move on to introducing combinations of flavours. Don't be afraid to include herbs and spices to introduce baby to lots of new tastes! Try also to include iron and vitamin C sources where possible. Some of the recipes in this book are also ideal for this stage, or you can blend up any of the other age-appropriate recipes you fancy.

SPOON-FED: AIM FOR LUMPIER TEXTURES

- Carrot, butternut squash & cumin
- Super-green Avocado Dip (see page 86)
- Broccoli & apple
- Berry Smoothie Bowl (see page 81)
- Coconut Lentil Dhal (see page 131)
- Spiced Nectarine Overnight Oats (see page 88)
- Cannellini bean, lemon & parsley
- Chicken & sweet potato (ensure chicken is cooked before blending)

FINGER FOODS

- Pulled Chicken Fajitas (see page 118)
- Toast fingers
- Homemade meatballs
- Spinach & Banana Pancakes (see page 171)
- Berry & Chia Seed Cookies (see page 175)
- Lentil & Courgette Fritters (see page 176)
- Rigatoni or orzo pasta with tomato sauce
- Fluffy Pancakes (see page 84)

INTRODUCING ALLERGENS

This is an important step when weaning for any parent, but when you're an allergy parent with a 'higher risk' baby I completely understand how scary it can feel to introduce allergens.

Although it's worrying, and you may feel like avoiding the risk of a reaction completely, research shows that excluding allergens from your child's diet until 12 months old may actually **increase** the risk of allergy.[18] So it's really important to tackle allergens, and preferably quite soon into your weaning journey, once baby is swallowing effectively (as you want to be confident that they have actually consumed the allergen). Personally, we started two weeks into weaning.

Ideally if you're higher risk, then introducing allergens would be guided by your dietitian, who can support you through the process. The guidance here covers the approach and 'how to' for the most common allergens and focuses on taking it slow and steady, which is particularly important when you already have atopic history.

Top allergens

The UK currently recognises these as the top 14 allergens, which must be highlighted on food packets. Those with a * are considered the **top nine**, which are the most prevalent in the UK and are the focus for introducing when weaning.

- Celery
- Cereals containing gluten (wheat*, rye, barley)
- Cow's milk*
- Crustaceans* (crab, lobster, prawns/shrimp, scampi)
- Eggs*
- Fish*
- Lupin (a legume sometimes found in flour and baked products)
- Molluscs (oysters, mussels, land snails, squid and whelks)
- Mustard
- Peanuts* (technically a legume, not a nut)
- Sesame*
- Soya*
- Sulphur dioxide (otherwise known as sulphites)
- Tree nuts* (almonds, Brazil nuts, cashews, hazelnuts, pecans, pistachios, macadamia nuts, walnuts)

> **Wheat and gluten are two different things!**
> This confuses a lot of people, so let's clear it up.
> **Wheat** = a cereal grain, which contains a range of proteins, one or more of which children can be allergic to.
> **Gluten** = a specific protein (the one that makes bread springy) found in wheat, but also in barley and rye.
> Coeliac disease is an autoimmune condition, not an allergy, but often causes confusion because it's caused by an adverse reaction to eating gluten. When someone with coeliac disease consumes gluten, it triggers an immune response that damages the lining of the small intestine. Symptoms in children can include diarrhoea, nausea/vomiting, bloating, extreme tiredness, nutrient deficiencies, e.g. iron and folate, and faltering growth. There is also a strong hereditary link, so if a direct family member has coeliac disease, it's much more likely for a child to have it too.

OTHER FOOD ALLERGIES

It's possible to be allergic to any foods. While the top 14 allergens are the most common, there seem to be others growing in prevalence, such as avocado, bananas, coconut, corn, kiwi, legumes (beans, lentils, chickpeas, peas), oats and tomato.

How to approach allergen introduction

Before you introduce an allergen, you must make sure that your baby is well, with any eczema under control (if struggling, seek advice from your GP or dermatologist).

Based on the advice I was given by healthcare professionals I've put together this **SSS** acronym as an easy way of remembering the general approach to introducing allergens:

Single - Introduce one single allergen at a time and wait three days between each one.
Small - Offer a very small amount the first time you introduce it.
Slow - Slowly build up the amount (assuming there's no reaction).

Introduce the allergen in the morning, so that you have the whole day to spot any potential reactions. You may also want to take a photo of baby's skin before you offer the meal, so it's easier to compare any potential reactions (e.g. a rash) to what's 'normal' for them.

Consider offering on weekdays, as in case of a reaction that needs medical attention there are more medical facilities open. Some people feel safer introducing allergens for the first time near the hospital (the car park seems to be a popular choice!). If it's somewhere you can have baby safely sitting in a highchair and harness, then go for it, but it's definitely not required! I personally always offered allergens at home but made sure I had my partner with me, and we had the change bag ready, in case we needed to get to the hospital quickly.

If you have been prescribed an antihistamine or Adrenaline Auto-Injector, have these prepared before you introduce allergens. I used to pre-measure Jude's antihistamine into a syringe ready just in case.

Once it's in, keep it in. So, once an allergen has been introduced successfully, this should be offered regularly in the diet (2-3 times per week) to maintain tolerance.

> **Lucy says:** *'When talking about introducing allergens to parents, I always reinforce that severe reactions like anaphylaxis during weaning are* **extremely rare**.*'*

How to introduce each allergen

The focus when weaning should be introducing the **top nine** individually, so here you'll find guidance on how to serve each of these (I've included cow's milk just in case you happen to be reading this and are not dairy free, but obviously don't introduce if they have CMPA!).

The recommended order to introduce is egg first, then peanut, then after that it's up to you.

For all allergens remember to **start small**. Prepare the allergen as per the guidance below, then offer in the following amounts:

Day 1 - ¼ tsp of the allergen as prepared below, then if tolerated;
Day 2 - ½ tsp, then if tolerated;
Day 3 - 1 tsp

The aim is to be confident that your baby has consumed the whole amount, so you may want to consider mixing with a food you know they like.

Allergens should be introduced directly through food. Lucy says: *'Don't be tempted to rub an allergen on to your child's skin first to "test" for any reaction. Many children would experience skin irritation or redness with this, completely unrelated to allergy. This is not an accurate way to expose a child to food allergens.'*

Remember as well as observing for immediate (IgE) reactions you're also observing for delayed (non-IgE) reactions up to 72 hours after consumption.

Egg - Boil an egg in boiling water for 15 minutes, leave to cool, then peel and mash in a bowl with some water or your child's milk. Mix with a soft food like mashed sweet potato or avocado. If tolerated after day 3, you can then try less well-cooked eggs, for example scrambled or an omelette.

Peanut - Mix smooth, 100% natural peanut butter with some water to loosen, then mix with mashed banana or porridge.

Cow's milk - Plain or Greek-style dairy yoghurt.

Crustacean - Cooked prawns diced or minced very finely and mixed with a soft food like mashed potato.

Fish - Use fresh fish fillet (rather than canned) and steam or poach so it's soft and mashable. Start with ¼ tsp mashed fish and mix it into mashed potato or avocado. If tolerated, you can then introduce other types of fish individually (remember to keep a food diary so you can note any reactions).

Sesame - Tahini (sesame seed paste) or hummus with tahini as an ingredient (see recipe on page 112). Mix with mashed banana or porridge.

Soya - Toasted bread with soya flour as an ingredient or plain soya yoghurt.

Tree nuts - Follow guidance for peanuts above, but for individual tree nuts. Use either a shop-bought nut butter (ensure it is 100% of the specific nut, not a blend) or buy the nuts whole and grind them to a fine paste in a food processor. Never offer nuts whole.

Wheat - Wheat biscuit cereal mixed with baby's usual milk until soft. If tolerated after day 3, you can introduce fingers of toast, and pasta.

For the remaining five top allergens you can absolutely introduce individually following the guidance above if you're worried. Keeping a food diary would be another way to identify a potential allergy if you had any concerns about reactions.

If there's no reaction following day 3, you can progress to amounts larger than a teaspoon, and remember to include them regularly in the diet to maintain tolerance.

What if there's a reaction?

While it can feel really scary before you introduce an allergen, the data is reassuring in that 998-999 babies out of 1,000 will not have a severe reaction to a food that's introduced.[19] It's important to be confident in what you're looking for when it comes to reactions, however, and remain vigilant.

IMMEDIATE SYMPTOMS (WITHIN 30 MINUTES OF CONSUMPTION):

- Swollen lips, face or eyes
- Hives or itchy skin rash
- Vomiting

Action: If not severe enough to suspect anaphylaxis, call 111 for advice.

DELAYED SYMPTOMS (UP TO 72 HOURS AFTER CONSUMPTION):

- Abdominal discomfort, vomiting, diarrhoea, mucus, or blood in stool
- Dry, itchy skin (eczema) or rash
- (Rarely) constipation

Action: Avoid giving the allergen again, take note of all symptoms and book an appointment to discuss with your GP.

CONTACT REACTION

Babies may get a red, spotty or blotchy rash, or patches of it, around their mouth, neck or hands after eating certain foods. This can cause concern for parents but is actually not a food allergy and rather the skin being irritated by the food. It can often be more noticeable in children with more sensitive skin, or eczema too. Common foods to cause this are:

- Tomatoes or tomato-based sauce
- Citrus fruits or acidic fruits like strawberries
- Foods rich in histamine, e.g. aubergine or spinach
- Spices or seasonings

It's more likely to be a contact reaction, rather than an allergy if:

- The rash is localised to where the food contact has taken place - so generally around the mouth/lips/face. NOT widespread, on their torso or raised.
- Should get better once washed gently/without any treatment, NOT get worse, spread or be combined with any other symptoms.
- Baby doesn't seem bothered by the rash. NOT seeming distressed.

Action: Consider applying a barrier cream (like petroleum jelly) around the mouth before offering the food again. If you're concerned, speak to a healthcare professional.

OTHER REACTIONS TO CONSIDER

If you suspect these make sure you discuss them with a healthcare professional.

FPIES (Food Protein Induced Enterocolitis Syndrome): a rare non-IgE mediated food allergy that affects the gastro-intestinal tract and typically causes significant vomiting, diarrhoea, lethargy and dehydration 1-4 hours after consumption of a food trigger. It doesn't cause skin or breathing issues. The most common food triggers are cow's milk, soya, grains, certain fruits or vegetables, and meat.

Oral allergy syndrome (aka Pollen food syndrome): A hypersensitivity reaction to certain fruits, vegetables and/or nuts causing irritant symptoms like itching, tingling or mild swelling of the mouth, lips and/or throat. This is caused when individuals who are allergic to certain pollens cross-react to these foods. It's very uncommon in young children, and most common in older children who have developed hay fever.

Anaphylaxis

While it's rare, and something no-one wants to think about happening to their child, it's really important to be aware of the signs of anaphylaxis and to know what to do if it happens. It's a serious allergic reaction which can be life threatening, so it always needs emergency treatment. Anaphylaxis only occurs in IgE mediated (immediate) allergies, however, not all IgE mediated allergies result in anaphylaxis.

Look out for the ABC symptoms:
Airways: Swelling in the throat, tongue or upper airways (tightening of the throat, hoarse voice or cry, difficulty swallowing).
Breathing: Sudden onset wheezing, breathing difficulty, noisy breathing.
Circulation: Dizziness, feeling faint, sudden sleepiness, tiredness, confusion, pale, clammy skin, loss of consciousness/floppiness.

Other symptoms may include:
- swelling of lips, face or eyes.
- raised hives.
- stomach pain/nausea/vomiting.

As babies and pre-verbal children will struggle to communicate symptoms, be aware of other signs such as scratching their face and neck, pulling ears, distress or unusual clinginess. Older children may say things like their mouth is 'itchy', 'tingly' or 'feels weird'.

If there are any signs of anaphylaxis:
- If you have an Adrenaline Auto-Injector (AAI), use it straight away. DO NOT DELAY.
- Immediately call 999, ask for an ambulance, say clearly '**anaphylaxis**' (*pronounced 'ana-fill-axis'*), then give precise details of your location including postcode.
- If they are not already, lie your child down with their legs raised.
- If there has been no improvement after five minutes, use their second AAI.

ADRENALINE AUTO-INJECTORS (AAIs)

AAIs are adrenaline injector devices designed for self-use, or in the case of a child, administered to them by an adult. Adrenaline (aka epinephrine) acts quickly to reverse the symptoms of anaphylaxis, opening up the airways by reducing swelling and raising blood pressure. To work effectively, it must be administered as soon as possible if there are any signs of anaphylaxis.

Anyone who is at risk of anaphylaxis should always carry **two** in-date AAIs with them at all times – there must also be two at any childcare setting they attend.

There are currently three brands of AAI available in the UK which are all available on prescription: EpiPen®, Jext® and Emerade®. All three have a set of instructions, and offer training devices to practise, so it's really important that you feel comfortable with how to use the one your child has been prescribed and ask for training from a healthcare professional. All three are administered into the middle of the outer thigh, through clothing if required.

Expiry and storage
The AAI dose is relevant to weight, so you'll need to be prescribed new devices as your child grows. Adrenaline degrades over time and may be less effective after the expiry date, so make sure you replace your AAIs before the expiry. You must also check your AAIs regularly to ensure the liquid is clear and colourless. If it seems discoloured or contains particles, you should replace it. If you think your AAIs look defective, return them immediately and report this using the MHRA's Yellow Card Scheme.[20]

Always check the storage instructions on the box, but generally it's advised to keep in the original packaging to prevent light exposure, to keep below 25°C and not to freeze. In hot weather, you'll need to think about storing the AAI in an insulated medical bag to avoid it overheating.

For lots more information and advice on anaphylaxis check out Anaphylaxis UK.

Allergy Parents' Guide to Life

When I started my allergy parent journey, I remember clearly just how much I worried about how to navigate key moments for the first time. Playdates. Nursery. Birthday parties. Holidays. Events that other parents were excited about filled me with dread. But I never wanted my children to miss out just because they had a food allergy, and we've successfully experienced all the things I was scared about. This chapter aims to support you with navigating your daily life, and the different milestones you'll face as your child grows.

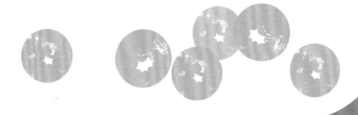

MY ALLERGY PARENT PRINCIPLES

1. Trust your instincts

If something doesn't feel right, **trust your gut**. I can't say it enough – a parent's intuition is powerful, and you know your child better than anyone else. If you're worried about something, get it checked out. Don't let anyone make you feel like you're being silly or overprotective.

2. Learn as much as you can

'Knowledge is power' as they say, and you've already taken the first step by reading this book! Learning the facts about CMPA will help give you the tools to inform others, and understanding about key nutrients will give you confidence in meeting your child's nutritional needs. My hope for everyone is that they have a supportive healthcare team, including a dietitian – if that's you, ask them lots of questions! If not, read the resources outlined in the back of this book, and make it your mission to be as informed as possible.

3. Set clear boundaries

Rules that you implement at home, and communicate to others, can help to ensure that everyone is working together effectively to keep your child safe. You can even pop these on the fridge so everyone can see them. Think about:

- Whether your child can eat 'may contains'.
- A hand washing regime before and after meals.
- Whether you will allow the allergen(s) into the house, and if so consider:
  - Setting rules about where it/they can be consumed.
  - Ensuring that areas used in food prep and eating are sanitised before and after, and that anyone involved in food prep washes their hands.
  - Having a different shelf in the fridge for products containing any of your child's allergens.
  - Ensuring plates, cutlery and cups are well cleaned before each use (or have separate colours if this works for you).

4. Be kind to yourself

Being an allergy parent is hard. It can feel relentless, overwhelming and exhausting. You may feel like you're on high alert all the time, never really getting a break from the worry or mental load of planning everything. So try not to beat yourself up too much if you have a wobble, or even if there's a slip-up (it happens!). Try to find a support network of families who are on the same journey, whether that's in person or online; having someone else who understands really helps. Be open with your partner/family/friends about any anxieties you are feeling – try not to keep things bottled up. Also, while I know most mums will laugh at this one, do try to get a break every now and again to do something just for you!

5. Prep, plan and pack

Organisation is crucial when you're an allergy parent (as sadly we don't really have the luxury of spontaneity!) The three Ps are a helpful tool to keep in your head:

PREP

Always have a safe stash of snacks in the cupboards and your bag, plus containers of safe meals in the freezer for when you can't be bothered to cook. Save recipes that your child likes (hint hint!) and send copies to family or childminders who make any of your child's meals.

PLAN

Thinking ahead is key. Consider setting aside a time every week (with your partner if relevant, and a tipple or a brew perhaps!) where you run through:

- Meal plan for the week ahead and create a shopping list.
- Childcare plans, appointments and any other logistical bits.
- Social occasions, including any communications you've had with the organiser and anything you need to organise or pack to cater for your child's allergies.

PACK

Create an allergy pack that you carry with you at all times, and also give one to any caregivers. This should contain:

- Allergy Action Plan if they are at risk of anaphylaxis, including their name, a photo and date of birth. This should detail what AAI they are prescribed, when and how it should be used, plus emergency contact details. There are templates for these available on the BSACI website to be completed by a healthcare professional.[21]
- If not at risk of anaphylaxis, consider an allergy alert card with their name, allergies and symptoms and what should be done if they have a reaction.
- Antihistamine/AAIs/inhaler/emollient if prescribed (ensure everything is in date).
- Sanitising wipes, reusable cloths and hand sanitiser.

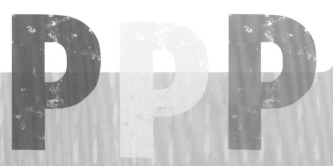

COMMUNICATION

Something I didn't include in my principles because it really deserves a section of its own, is communication. For me, good communication is the most important tool in an allergy parent's journey.

Communicating with others

Before your child can advocate for themselves, they'll rely on you to be their voice. I find these considerations helpful:

- **Be understanding.** Remember that many people won't have experience of food allergies nor know a lot about them. Try to be empathetic to that and to start from a place of wanting to help them understand.

- **Be clear and direct.** e.g. 'My child is allergic to cow's milk. If he eats any, he will get an itchy rash, painful tummy and diarrhoea. This includes dairy products like cheese, yoghurt and ice cream but also any product with cow's milk as an ingredient.' Avoid vague language like 'he can't really have dairy'.

- **Be prepared to educate.** Don't assume that people will automatically understand what ingredients would trigger your child's food allergy - some people confuse dairy and eggs for example, or wheat and gluten. Many also confuse CMPA with lactose intolerance, so don't be afraid to correct them and explain the difference.

- **Stay calm.** Perhaps this is easier said than done in certain circumstances, but trying to keep calm when having important conversations can help you speak logically and be solution oriented. If a conversation feels hard face to face or at the time, come back to it or think about other ways to communicate, e.g. a voice note, or email.

- **Don't be afraid to speak up.** If you feel that you're being dismissed, or you're asking for support but not getting it, be persistent! I've grown to not really care if I'm considered difficult or pushy if the outcome is important.

Dealing with unhelpful opinions

Unfortunately, it's likely you'll be confronted with a few opinionated people and infuriating comments in the course of your allergy journey. Some I've heard include:

'I'm sure a little bit wouldn't hurt.'
'Can't you just scrape the cheese off?'
'Give them it enough and they'll get used to it.'
'Ahhh, you're a first-time mum, aren't you?'
'We didn't have all these "allergies" in my day.'
'Oh, what a shame they can't have chocolate.'

If you hear these, I'm sure your blood will be boiling. Try to remember, though, that most of these comments come from a place of unawareness and not understanding, rather than intending to be hurtful. So try to be patient and use it as an opportunity to inform. If it's someone involved in your child's life (rather than a nosy stranger) and they're really struggling to get their head around it, give them this book! Or signpost them to the resources mentioned at the back.

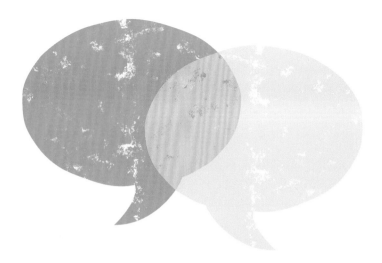

Communicating with your child

Hopefully, your child will outgrow their food allergies. However, if they don't, it's important that you are teaching them the skills they'll need to manage their allergy independently when they're older. I really believe that it's never too early to be talking about your child's allergies with them. From the beginning, even before they can talk, your child will absorb a lot more than you realise, and it's also helpful for any siblings to see and hear. Be aware that children pick up on your tone and body language, so try to consider how you talk about things so as not to scare them.

- Openly discuss their food allergies and what symptoms they get, in language they might understand, e.g. 'peanuts are not safe for you to eat, they make you sick and give you a poorly tummy.'
- Role model checking labels, narrate out loud what you're looking for and why it's safe: 'I'm checking for milk in bold on the ingredients list. Look – it's not there, you can eat this!'
- Explain and role model the basics of what they should do to keep themselves safe:
  - Washing hands before and after meals.
  - Only eating food that's for them (not sharing or stealing food), or prompting them to come and ask you if they can have it.
  - Saying 'no thank you, I have food allergies' if they're offered food that you're not sure is safe.
  - Using only their own tableware and cutlery.
  - Always letting an adult know if they've touched or consumed their food allergen.

- Talk about upcoming appointments or hospital visits, chat through what will happen and role play with teddies or a doctor's kit.
- Explain what happens in an emergency and why, for example if an AAI is used, what this does, and how it might make them feel.
- Encourage them to be open with their feelings if they feel excluded, upset or anxious so you can support them.

When age-appropriate you can then look to teach them:

- How to recognise their symptoms. Some children might think 'my tongue feels fuzzy' or 'I feel weird' without realising this is a reaction, so it's important to encourage them to say something to an adult the minute something doesn't feel quite right in their body.
- The emergency process, including how to administer their AAI (you can practise using a training device).
- How to order at restaurants and ask questions about how meals are prepared.
- How to cook and prepare their favourite meals and snacks.

CHECKING LABELS

Shopping as an allergy parent can feel so overwhelming at first. Before you were dairy free, the chances are that you never really looked at the back of packets, or worried about the ingredients when ordering a takeaway. I certainly didn't! But suddenly it will become a huge part of your life. While it can feel daunting at first, I promise that in time you will become a labels expert, scanning ingredients quickly and confidently.

The first thing to say is that it's absolutely crucial to check the ingredients of everything. **EVERYTHING**! I'm still constantly surprised by the number of products that cow's milk can sneak into, such as stock cubes, gravy and crisps. Don't assume it's only food you need to check either – toiletries, creams and even teething powder can also contain allergens. Frustratingly, manufacturers can, and do, change the ingredients of products, so even if it's something you buy regularly, the golden rule is:

> **Always check the ingredients on the pack, every single time.**
> In the UK, the current law states that for pre-packaged foods, any of the top 14 allergens present in the ingredients are highlighted **in bold**, *italics*, highlighted or **in a different font** on the packet ingredients. This includes if it's a variation of the allergen (e.g. whey powder, **from milk**).

WHAT'S THE DEAL WITH 'MAY CONTAINS'?

Urgh, the dreaded Precautionary Allergen Labelling (PAL). These statements confuse a lot of people, and for good reason. You'll see a range of phrases that all effectively mean the same thing, like:

'May contain traces of'
'Cannot guarantee there are no traces of'
'Not suitable for allergy sufferers'
'Made in a factory which...'

What this means is that there's a risk of cross-contamination due to the manufacturing process. For example, a biscuit that does not have cow's milk in the ingredients is made on the same production line as another biscuit which does. So there's a risk that a trace of cow's milk is transferred, contaminating the milk-free biscuit.

Surprisingly, in the UK there is currently no legal requirement to use PAL. The guidance for companies is that they should only use PAL when there is a 'genuine risk of cross-contamination identified which, following a risk assessment, cannot be removed through risk management actions'. However, it is ultimately the decision of the company whether to include one on their packs or not.

INGREDIENTS

Lemon Filling (50%) (Sugar, Cocoa Butter, Coconut Milk, Rice Flour, Glucose Syrup, Lemon Juice, Water, Flavouring, Emulsifiers: Sunflower Lecithin, Mono- and Diglycerides of Fatty Acids, Sucrose Esters of Fatty Acids, Palm Oil, Rapeseed Oil, Fructose, Cornflour, Dextrose, Acidity Regulators: Citric Acid, Sodium Citrate; Concentrated Lemon Juice, Preservative: Potassium Sorbate; Colour: Lutein; Humectant: Glycerine; Salt, Lemon Oil, Rice Starch), Rice Flour, Tapioca Starch, Palm Oil, Oligofructose, Rapeseed Oil, Sugar, Water, Ground **Almonds**, Glucose, Salt, Thickener: Xanthan Gum; Colour: Plain Caramel; Cornflour, Emulsifier: Mono- and Diglycerides of Fatty Acids.

For allergens, see ingredients in **bold**. Made in an environment that handles other nuts and egg. May contain traces of peanut.

ADDITIONAL INFO

Suitable for vegans. Suitable for coeliacs.

Made in our dedicated gluten, wheat and milk free bakery.

INGREDIENTS

Mincemeat (42%) (Sugar, Apple Purée, Sultanas, Raisins, Glucose Syrup, Currants, Brandy, Palm Oil, Glucose-Fructose Syrup, Orange Peel, Rice Flour, Cinnamon, Acidity Regulators (Acetic Acid, Citric Acid), Coriander, Lemon Peel, Sunflower Oil, Ginger, Caraway, Treacle, Orange Oil], Rice Flour, Tapioca Flour, Palm Oil, Brown Sugar, Sugar, Rapeseed Oil, **Almonds**, Dextrose, Salt, Thickener (Xanthan Gum), Cornflour, Emulsifier (Mono- and Diglycerides of Fatty Acids).

Allergy Advice
For allergens, see ingredients in **bold**. Also, may contain peanuts and other nuts.

Prepared to a vegan recipe, not suitable for egg allergy sufferers because this allergen is present in the environment.

Gluten Free, Wheat Free, Milk Free.

Ingredients

Wheat flour, palm oil, sugar, glucose-fructose syrup, raising agents (calcium phosphates, ammonium carbonates, sodium carbonates, potassium carbonates), salt, **barley** malt flour. **May contain egg, milk.**

Suitable for vegetarians

For best before date, see base of box. Some settling of contents may have occurred during transport.

Can you or your child consume 'may contain' products?

Unfortunately, there's no easy answer to this, and simply, it's so child-dependent that it's always best to get individualised advice from your healthcare professional. This is because it depends on a few factors, including the severity of the allergy and the level of risk that parents feel comfortable with. This is a personal choice and will be different from family to family, so in part it may come down to what feels best for **you**.

If you are dealing with an IgE mediated allergy and/or your child is considered to be at high risk of anaphylaxis, then you may be advised to avoid them completely. Personally, I give Jude (who has delayed CMPA) 'may contain' products and, touch wood, we've never had an issue. If you're able to tolerate them, then it does open up a lot more options for foods, but it's a personal decision.

FREE FROM PRODUCTS

If a product is labelled 'free-from' milk, then that is a guarantee the product is milk-free – both in its ingredients and also it not being at risk of cross-contamination. Vegan products do not fall under this rule, so a food can be labelled 'vegan' but have a PAL for milk.

NATASHA'S LAW

Following campaigning by the parents of Natasha Ednan-Laperouse after her heartbreaking death from anaphylaxis (after eating a baguette without sesame seeds labelled on the packaging), Natasha's Law came into effect in the UK in October 2021. This changed the legalities of PPDS – foods which are prepacked for direct sale or food that is packaged at the same place it is offered or sold to consumers and is in this packaging before it is ordered or selected. The law now states that **all** food outlets must provide full ingredient lists and clear allergen labelling for all food items.

LESSONS I'VE LEARNED

- Always trust your gut – if you don't understand a packet's label, or feel uneasy about the information you're being given, avoid.
- Personally, I think ordering food online always presents a slight risk, especially via third party apps, in that you're trusting that the takeaway has updated the allergen information on their sites. I always call the restaurant to go through each dish and its ingredients, and if I don't feel confident, then I don't order.
- Be aware that some cosmetics use Latin names for certain ingredients, including nuts. Lists of these are available online.
- Some supermarket websites and apps allow you to filter products by allergens you avoid, which is really handy – just remember to always double check the pack in person, as updates can sometimes be missed.
- Sign up to Food Standards Agency (FSA) allergy alerts, which pings you an email whenever there is a recall due to incorrect product labelling relating to your allergy.

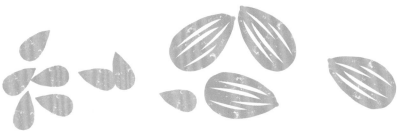

CHILDCARE

I know that childcare is probably the biggest area of worry for a lot of you. As parents all we want is to keep our children safe, healthy and happy, and it's so important that you feel comfortable with whoever is looking after them.

Your child with food allergies has needs, which have to be clearly understood and appreciated by caregivers. They must also feel like they can handle the responsibility. It may be upsetting for someone to say 'no' but you must also respect that decision, as ultimately the most important thing is the safety of your child.

Choosing childcare is a big decision, and I've put together the below tips to ensure that you feel as prepared as possible.

Family, friends and babysitters
(Non-professional childcare)

- Organise a meeting with them ahead of their first time looking after your child, at a time that you can both give it your full attention.
- Make sure they understand what your child can and can't eat, how to check labels and how to prepare food safely.
- Explain how to recognise a reaction and what to do if this happens. Go through your child's Allergy Action Plan if they have one, including the emergency procedure. Teach them how to store and administer any medications, in particular an AAI if this is needed, having them practise in front of you so you're confident they would be able to use it if needed.
- Ask if they can 'shadow' you for a few hours when you're looking after your child so they can get a better understanding of the processes you follow for their allergies.
- Empower them with helpful info - provide recipes, advice, give them a stash of allergy-friendly snacks or offer to provide meals for them if they would prefer.
- Hand over an *allergy pack* (see page 57) and run through the contents, plus tableware, cutlery, bibs and anything else they might need.
- Agree how they'll update you throughout the day, including if there are any suspected reactions. I've always used the mantra '*Text if good, call if bad*' so I knew if I got a call that it was something I needed to talk to them about straight away.
- If a slip up happens, chat it through with them afterwards to figure out what went wrong, and how you can make sure it's avoided next time.

Nursery, childminders and school
(Professional childcare)

Any registered childcare setting or individual has a duty of care to safeguard and promote the welfare of your child.[22] While this is reassuring, as a parent you'll no doubt want to dig into the details of exactly how your child will be kept safe. Often, you'll leave a visit and have a gut feeling either way of whether a setting is right for your child, but it's helpful to be structured about your visits and consider several options.

Request a private meeting with the management team to talk through the details of your child's allergies, their Allergy Action Plan if relevant and share any worries you have. Ask lots of questions about their allergy policies and procedures, for example:

- Do they allow food from outside the setting to be brought in? If so, are there any restrictions?
- How do they identify children with allergies (e.g. do they have photos/allergy information displayed?) and how are staff informed of this, including any supply staff?
- What steps do they take during mealtimes and snacks to prevent a child coming into contact with their food allergen?
- Are any allergens used outside of food times, i.e. during play or lessons? If so, are these sessions adapted to support inclusion?
- What is the staff training policy, including AAI training?
- How and where is medication stored?
- Example food menus, so you can get a sense of what your child would be eating, or how they tailor menus for allergens.
- What milk alternatives are offered? Are these provided by the setting or do parents need to provide them?
- Do they ever have food distributed as treats, rewards or celebrations, e.g. class prizes/birthdays?

Ask yourself these three questions when evaluating the options after your visits:

1. Do they have clear processes? (i.e. do you understand the steps they would take to avoid an allergic reaction and do you feel reassured that they would know what to do if there was a reaction?)
2. Was their communication clear, open and did it provide you with confidence?
3. Did you get a gut feel that the team there would do everything they can to keep your child safe and happy?

Once you've selected a setting

When it gets closer to the time of your child starting, ask for another meeting with the management team to discuss the specifics of your child's food allergy.

- Run through their Allergy Action Plan again.
- Hand over medication for your child. If they are prescribed an AAI, you will need to give them two. Agree where this will be stored, and think about different circumstances, e.g. classroom-based work, sports, trips etc.
- Agree communication lines for what happens in case of emergency and if there is a possibility your child has come into contact with their food allergen.
- Decide whether your child will be having a packed lunch or whether the setting will cater for them. If the latter, it's helpful for the setting's representative to be at that meeting and run through specifics of meal and snack times, e.g. what exactly what will be offered, how cross-contamination will be avoided (if relevant).

You may also want to consider:

- Requesting that parents are advised about your child's allergies and that food is limited from being brought into the setting.
- Offering to do a talk for staff with a refresher on administering an AAI if relevant.
- Giving staff a stash of safe treats for any occasions when food may be distributed to the class.

What to do if you have a complaint
If something has gone wrong, or you're not happy that the processes are being followed, it's important to discuss it with the setting as soon as possible. Request a meeting with the management team/childminder to outline your concerns and give them the opportunity to respond. Try to be constructive with the end goal of agreeing 'How can we prevent this happening again?' If the problem is not resolved, or it needs escalating, follow the setting's formal complaint procedure. Should you still have a concern afterwards, you can complain to the Department of Education or Ofsted.

GOING OUT TO EAT

If the thought of going to a restaurant with your child makes you nervous, I totally get it! Handing over control of food prep to strangers, especially if you're dealing with severe or multiple allergies, can be a tricky thing to get your head around.

Going out to eat is absolutely possible – the key is doing your research and planning ahead. In my personal experience, some of the larger chains (I'm going to shout out wagamama, Nando's, Ask Italian and Pizza Express here) have good allergy policies, with steps like a manager always taking your order and food arriving clearly marked with allergy stickers. That doesn't mean there aren't lots of excellent independent and smaller restaurants that you'll be able to enjoy.

In the UK, restaurants are currently required by law to give allergy information in writing, either with:

- Allergy information written on the menu or in a book/pack.
- A clearly visible notice explaining how customers can get this information (e.g. for allergy information, please speak directly to your waiter).
- For buffets, the information needs to be for each individual food, not as a whole.

If you are buying takeaway, food online or over the phone, you have the right to be provided with allergen information before purchase, either in writing or over the phone. Then again at the point of delivery, so by stickers on the food for example.

How to manage restaurant visits

PLAN WHERE YOU GO

- Check out the restaurant website and menus they have online – they may even have a separate allergy menu.
- Search for reviews on TripAdvisor® that mention the words 'allergy' or 'dairy free'.
- Consider booking the table at a time outside of peak service hours, as you will hopefully get more access to staff and the kitchen during your visit if needed.

LET THE RESTAURANT KNOW

- Add a note to the booking to let them know about the allergy.
- If it would make you feel more comfortable, call the restaurant at a quiet time, speak to the manager, and ask about their allergy procedures and what safe dishes they could offer – you'll soon get a sense of whether they take it seriously or not.

PACK A BAG

- Always ensure you have your *allergy pack* (see page 57).
- Pack a bib, cutlery, plate and water cup that only your child uses. This can help reduce the anxiety over possible cross-contamination.
- Make sure you've packed a back-up meal/snack option in case there's an issue.

ON ARRIVAL

- Make sure the server looking after you, and the manager if appropriate, knows about the allergy and understands what this means they have to avoid. You may also want to show them and the chef your child's allergy alert card.
- Thoroughly clean down the highchair/chair, table and any mats situated near your child's seat.

ASK (LOTS OF) QUESTIONS

- Don't be afraid to ask, even if you feel like 'that annoying customer' - it's important that you feel comfortable!
- Ask for the allergy book or information.
- If you're dealing with a severe allergy, ask about how the food is prepared and any risks of cross-contamination (e.g. is the food cooked in the same fryer as products containing the allergen?). Ask to speak to the chef if that would help.
- If you don't feel totally comfortable once your questions have been answered, use your back-up meal if necessary.

CONSIDER YOUR OWN CHOICES

- Depending on the age of your child, think about whether they are going to try to steal food from someone else's plate or get upset because they want what you're eating. You may want to ensure all food is safe to avoid this.
- When Violet was a toddler, I used to order a bowl of chips as an extra side (I asked for no salt to be added) so that she could have a couple and feel like she was eating the same as Mummy and not missing out.

WHEN THE FOOD ARRIVES

- Verbally confirm the dish you've ordered with the server when it arrives.
- Make sure you feel confident it's correct - sometimes you might just have a feeling it's not right, so don't be afraid to speak up and double check if that's the case. If in doubt - avoid.

IF THERE'S AN ISSUE

- The priority is the health and safety of your child, so focus the attention on them and follow your Allergy Action Plan if you have one.
- When the situation is under control, alert the manager and let them know as soon as possible.

AFTER YOUR VISIT

- If you've had an issue, or think things could have been better, take the time to send written feedback to the restaurant. Similarly if you were impressed or had a great experience, let the restaurant know; I'm sure it'll make someone's day.
- Make a note of where you've eaten, what your child ate and how you'd rate your experience so you have a reference for next time you're going out to eat.
- Write a review, share on forums or social media - I find that allergy parents always love reading about others' experiences, whether good or bad.

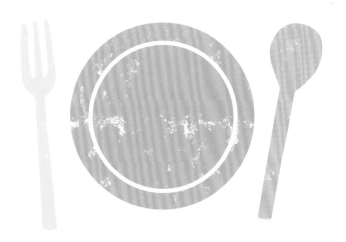

PARTIES, PLAYDATES AND SOCIAL OCCASIONS

One of the biggest struggles allergy parents face is wanting their child to enjoy social occasions without feeling like they're 'different' or 'excluded'. Being cautious and planning the details can really help increase your confidence in these situations.

When you're a guest

It's possible that the hosts won't have personally experienced food allergies, but I've found that the vast majority will be happy to take steps to make their event inclusive for your child.

It may feel awkward, but having a chat with the host before the event is really helpful. If you don't know them that well, try sending a message like:

'Dylan's so excited for Rosie's birthday, thanks so much for the invite! I wanted to let you know that he has an allergy to cow's milk and can't have any products with milk as an ingredient. Would you have time for a quick chat about the party so I can help cater for him?'

Then when you get the chance to talk:

- Explain about their food allergies and what reaction they have.
- Ask what food will be served, including cake and any items in party bags, and check if there's anything suitable. If not, ask if you can provide a safe version of the same food so your child feels included (you could get your child to pick their own so they feel excited).
- Explain that you'll need to sanitise their seat and table.
- Offer to stay with your child (depending on the type of occasion).

Remember to always pack a bag with the essentials, including their *allergy pack* (see page 57) back-up food and treats, tableware, bibs and water cup.

Always be appreciative of the efforts your hosts have gone to and say a big thank you afterwards. They may have been worried about 'getting it right', so this will mean a lot!

SOFT PLAY/ENTERTAINMENT VENUES

Play centres can be a real worry for allergy parents, because although most have rules about no food being consumed in the play areas, in my experience this is often not policed. If you're dealing with a severe allergy where you cannot risk cross-contamination, this can be tricky with ball pits, shared equipment etc.

- Speak to the management to let them know about your child's food allergy ahead of time and ask about their allergy policies, including how they will prevent food from being taken into the play areas.
- Ask about their cleaning schedules – it might be that you select a visit first thing in the morning when the venue has just been cleaned.
- Bring sanitising wipes and clean down as much as possible before your child plays.
- Ask if you can bring your own food (some of these venues have strict 'no food from outside' policies but may make exceptions for severe allergies).

When you're a host

Always communicate your child's food allergies ahead of time and ask parents to ensure that no outside food or drink containing the allergen is brought with them. Ask your guests about other food allergies, as it may be that you have multiple to consider. If so, you'll want to be proactive about making the event inclusive for them.

Consider creating labels/signs for each food on offer with allergens and may contains highlighted. I've previously prepared individual food bags with the guest's name and any allergies written on the bag to keep things simple.

Check out my party food recipes (see page 192) for lots of allergy-friendly food you can prepare.

HALLOWEEN TIP

If you'd like to go trick or treating, make a rule that no food can be eaten without your supervision, and tell your child in advance about the 'Switch Witch'. Any treats that they are given which contain dairy, put outside your house that night and in the morning the Switch Witch will have swapped them for safe alternatives or a toy!

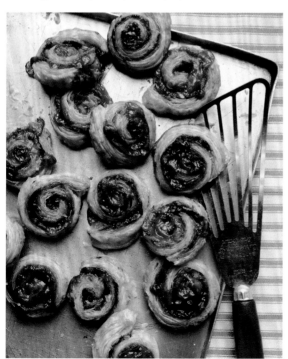

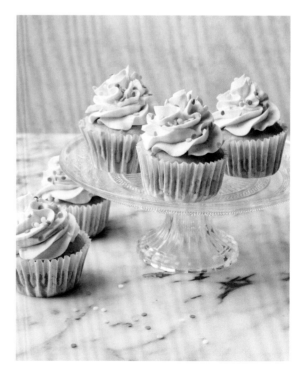

GOING ON HOLIDAY

Everyone deserves a holiday, none more so than allergy parents! If you're thinking about booking something for the first time, planning ahead can help alleviate some of the anxiety you might be feeling. Once you've decided the basics of whether you're going abroad or staying in the UK, and whether you're choosing a resort or going self-catering, you can get organised effectively by taking these practical steps.

Choosing accommodation

- Do a search for facilities in the local area, including restaurants, supermarkets and hospitals/doctors' surgeries to make sure there's everything you may need within a reasonable distance.
- If choosing a resort, search for keywords on reviews such as 'allergy', 'allergies' and 'dairy' to filter relevant reviews and insights from other families with allergies. You could also email the resort to ask questions about their allergy policies before you book.
- Check that the accommodation has a fridge if you'll need it for a milk alternative.

Flying

- Contact your airline before you fly, as many will offer extra luggage allowance for medical items.
- Check the airline's policy for bringing any milk alternatives/formula/medication you will need in hand luggage – most will allow this to be scanned separately at security and allowed as carry-on if proof of prescription or a doctor's note is shown.
- If food is offered on the aircraft, look at the options to see whether it will be suitable – some airlines do vegan meals, but most will be tailored for adults, so you may want to organise your own meals when travelling.
- Wipe down the seat, tray tables and window shutters with sanitising wipes.
- Let the cabin crew know about your child's food allergies.

Packing

- Check the expiration date for their medication before you pack it.
- Pack enough formula/plant-based milk alternative for your whole stay, plus some spare, in case of delays.
- Always pack lots of safe snacks and, assuming they are in sturdy packaging, some other basic items that could create easy meals, e.g. their favourite breakfast cereal, and a couple of jars or cartons of sauce you know they like.
- Other items to remember:
  - their *allergy pack* (see page 57)
  - food containers and bags
  - their own cutlery, plate/bowl and bibs
  - washing-up liquid, cleaning cloths/brushes for bottles and tableware

At a hotel

- Make the management team aware of allergies, and if possible, ask to speak to the chef or head of catering. They will be able to explain how food is labelled and may be able to make separate dishes on request.
- Remember to sanitise the seat and table before each meal.

Going abroad

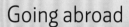

- Bear in mind that other countries have different approaches to food allergies, for example in terms of labelling laws, so look up how it works there so you're prepared.
- Consider getting allergy alert cards, and a copy of your child's Allergy Action Plan translated into the local language.
- Download Google Translate™ for scanning menus and ingredients.
- Practise the pronunciation of the allergens and note down how to say simple phrases such as 'My child is allergic to milk – does this contain milk?'
- Ensure you have reputable travel insurance and that any allergies are declared as a medical condition when you purchase it.

part two

let's cook!

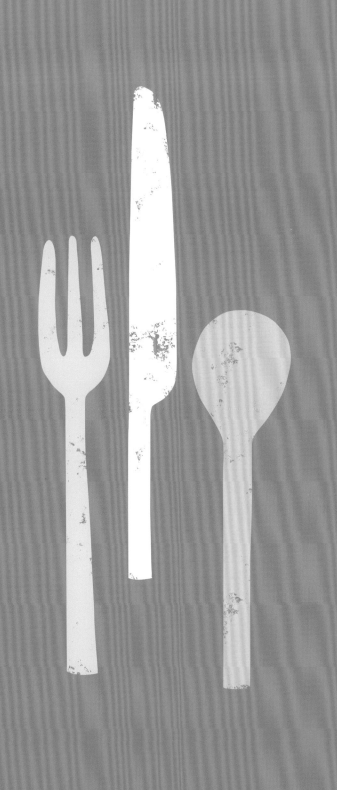

INGREDIENTS & ALTERNATIVES

Before we get into the recipes, here's a guide to the ingredients you'll always find stocked in my kitchen.

Dairy alternatives

Although I curse the cost, I'm always amazed at the constantly increasing range of dairy-free products on the shelves these days. A few years ago, there were only a handful, now there are hundreds!

BUTTER ALTERNATIVES/MARGARINE

Lots of margarine products are actually dairy free as they are usually made from vegetable oils (check individual pack labels). Any brand is suitable for use in my recipes and on toast, in sandwiches etc. You can also buy butter alternative and baking blocks; opt for the unsalted versions.

CHEESE ALTERNATIVES (CHEEZE)

OK, let's be real for a second… No, plant-based cheeze doesn't really taste like the dairy version, and the smell can take some getting used to! I'm still not a huge fan of eating it raw, but when you find one that melts well, it really does work nicely in recipes.

Cheeze that is currently available in the UK is usually coconut oil-based, and some brands contain other allergens including soya, gluten and nuts. Be aware that not all cheese alternatives are fortified with calcium, so choose one that is, and it's an added bonus if it has iodine and/or vitamin B12 too. It's good to be conscious of salt levels; a lot of cheeze products contain quite high amounts of salt, and these will count towards your child's daily salt limits (see page 35).

'Cheddar' cheeze – If you want to achieve a good 'melt' for pizza, toasties, lasagne etc, my advice is to buy a block (vs. pre-grated) and grate it finely using a Microplane grater rather than a standard cheese grater. Cooking low and slow works better than a high heat, and less is usually more.

'Mozzarella' cheeze – Generally available pre-grated. I've tried a lot, and I haven't yet found one that melts as well as 'Cheddar' cheeze grated finely. It will probably come down to whether you prefer the taste, as some can be milder than 'Cheddar' cheeze.

Soft/'cream' cheeze – There's been a big influx of new ones hitting the market recently, with lots of the big brands and supermarkets launching plant-based versions. You can also get flavoured versions such as garlic and herb, or chive.

Individual cheeze – A couple of brands now do individual calcium-fortified cheezes, which can be a nice addition for kids' lunchboxes or on-the-go; just be aware of salt levels.

Speciality cheeze – Ooh, fancy! Products I've spied on the shelves include alternatives to feta, Parmesan, crumbly blue, halloumi, Camembert and more, so do experiment and you may just find something that you and your family love.

> # Don't forget the golden rule:
> ## 'always check the ingredients on the pack, every time'.

CHOCOLATE

If you're a chocolate lover like me, and suddenly dairy free, you may be mourning the loss of your favourite treat! Don't forget though that chocolate in its pure form is dairy and egg free, as it's made from cocoa solids, cocoa butter (fat extracted from cocoa bean, not dairy butter) and sugar. So dark chocolate tends to be dairy free (always check!), but milk chocolate has cow's milk protein added. There are loads of milk chocolate alternatives available now, and several are allergy friendly and free from soya, gluten and nuts too. So try a few and you'll find a favourite for when you need a choccy fix.

CREAM ALTERNATIVES

Oat, soya or coconut cream alternatives can help add richness and creaminess to dishes, as well as being an accompaniment to puddings. You can also now find alternatives for crème fraîche, whipping cream and even canned spray cream.

CUSTARD ALTERNATIVES

There are a few refrigerated options available, across soya, oat and coconut varieties. You may also be surprised to learn that the leading brand of custard powder is actually dairy and egg free (may contain), so you can easily make custard with your favourite plant-based milk alternative.

MILK ALTERNATIVES

See page 41 for advice on choosing a plant-based milk alternative for children. For the recipes in this book, I've tended to use oat milk, but any milk alternative will work. You may find you prefer certain milk alternatives for different recipes - some are more savoury in flavour (pea, for example) whereas some are sweeter and work well in baking (e.g. soya, coconut).

YOGHURT ALTERNATIVES

Plain versions are best for babies and children - you can always sweeten them with fruit. I like to use the Greek-style ones in my recipes for a creamier result (available in oat, soya or coconut brands). Check they're fortified with calcium, and ideally iodine. Small, flavoured pots and pouches targeted at kids are available, but be aware of sugar levels. One idea is to buy reusable pouches online and fill them from a large pot with fruit mixed in.

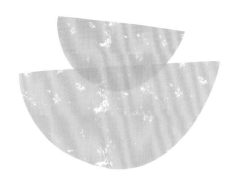

Storecupboard staples

BEANS AND PULSES (LEGUMES)

Cans of beans (white, black and red), chickpeas and bags of lentils are really nutritious staples to have in the cupboard. They're low-cost ingredients to bulk out meals or to provide a good source of protein and iron, especially if you're vegetarian, vegan or plant-based. Legume allergies are on the rise, so where there is an alternative in my recipes this is noted in the 'Top tips'.

BREAD

Most sliced bread is dairy free (always check!), as are lots of bagels, pitta and wraps. Soya free can be more challenging, as soya flour is a common bread ingredient, but there are options in both branded and supermarket own loaves. In the UK, flour used for white and brown bread needs to be fortified with calcium and iron by law, and some contain extra vitamins and minerals, so it can be a handy way of meeting nutrient requirements.

BREAKFAST CEREALS

Opt for well-fortified (calcium and iron) and low-sugar versions, for example wheat biscuits or multigrain hoops. Many of the supermarket own brands are nutritionally similar to the big brands, but not all - so always check the nutritional advice on the pack.

CHIA SEEDS

My favourite small but mighty nutrient booster! Packed with protein, calcium, healthy fats and more - stir into porridge and yoghurt, as well as using in my recipes. They're suitable from six months - you can grind or buy pre-ground (milled) but serving whole is fine as long as they're soaked in something 'wet'. Just be mindful of fibre content when giving to little ones (high fibre foods can fill up babies and young children before they've consumed enough energy and nutrients) - ½ teaspoon per portion is generally enough.

DESICCATED COCONUT

Violet calls it 'coconut sprinkles', so that's what it'll always be known as in our house! It's actually dried out, grated coconut flesh; a small amount in porridge, a smoothie or yoghurt alternative adds fibre and fat (a key nutrient for young children), as well as its delicious flavour.

GARLIC AND GINGER PASTES

I'm all for fresh ingredients, but when you just can't be bothered to chop, these pastes are brilliant to have handy.

HERBS AND SPICES

Crucial for adding flavour, especially when not adding salt. A well-stocked spice cupboard brings me a lot of joy! Don't be afraid of spices when cooking for babies and young children; it's a great way to introduce them to different tastes - just avoid chilli and cayenne pepper.

NUTRITIONAL YEAST (ALSO KNOWN AS NOOCH OR YEAST FLAKES)

It may look and smell like fish food, but I swear this is a game changer for dairy-free cooking! It adds a cheesy, savoury flavour to dishes, and it also has some vitamins, such as B12. As well as working nicely in creamy pasta and risotto, you can also sprinkle it on to mashed potato, soups or casseroles. Find it in the vegan aisle or near the stock cubes in bigger supermarkets, health food shops, or online. Some brands are 'may contain', so shop around for one suitable for you.

NUT BUTTERS

If nuts are tolerated, nut butters are a great way to include healthy fats and iron in your family's diet. Opt for smooth versions that are 100% nuts with no added sugar or salt. Be aware that even smooth versions can be quite thick, and you may need to loosen with some warm water if not adding to a warm dish. Always avoid offering directly off a spoon as this poses a choking risk.

OATS

Such a nutritious staple – as well as using them for porridge, I use them a lot in baking. I buy a large, cheap bag of porridge oats as they last ages. When weaning, you can whizz them up dry before using for a finer texture if preferred. Lots of 'baby cereal' brands contain milk, but many ready oats are only a 'may contain'; these can be a good option if tolerated as they're packed with vitamins and minerals.

OILS

I always have olive, coconut and vegetable oils stocked, plus spray bottle versions, and mix up what I use, generally preferring coconut oil for sweet recipes and curries, and olive or vegetable for more savoury dishes. However, to make the recipes in the book as allergy inclusive as possible, any oil can be used.

PACKAGED SNACKS

One I get asked about a lot – the reality is that when you don't have time to cook, or the freezer stash is empty, it's handy to have things in the cupboard that are easy to grab. I always have breadsticks, plain crackers and oat bars. For older children, I also have raisins and dried fruit shapes – be aware that the natural sugars in dried fruit can contribute to tooth decay, which is hugely on the rise for children, so keep limited or risk a telling off from the dentist!

PASSATA

I use passata (sieved tomatoes) in recipes over canned, chopped tomatoes when I want a smoother texture.

PASTA, RICE AND NOODLES

My favourite staples to create meals around. Quick-cook pasta and microwave rice pouches can be such a helpful time-saver if you're busy.

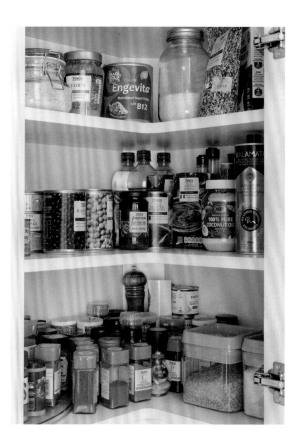

STOCK CUBES

If cooking for babies and young children, choose the low-salt or zero-salt versions (these are often soya free too, which some of the regular ones aren't).

XANTHAN GUM

You'll spot this in some of my recipes for a gluten-free adaptation – it's an additive that helps to improve the texture of GF baking in particular, making it less crumbly.

Freezer

VEG PACKS

Such a time-saver when it comes to recipe prep! I usually have chopped onions, leeks, peppers, sweet potato, spinach, sweetcorn and peas stocked, plus some packs of frozen herbs.

FRUIT

Really handy for stirring into porridge, whizzing up in smoothies or using in baking. Raspberries and mango chunks are our favourites, but you can also get large mixed bags of 'wonky' berries for a great value price.

FISH

Plain fish fillets can usually be steamed or baked straight from frozen, so can offer a quick meal solution – and we also always have cod or haddock fish fingers (a great source of iodine).

READY-ROLLED PUFF PASTRY

I was amazed to discover when I first went dairy free that most brands don't actually contain milk! Keep a couple of packs in the freezer ready to defrost for Pizza Pinwheels (see page 194) or PBJ Twists (see page 168).

Substitutes

When I post recipes, I'm often asked about substitutions, not just for the top allergens but some more uncommon ones. Here's a handy guide of alternatives you can refer to both for the recipes in this book, and elsewhere. Sometimes it takes a bit of trial and error when substituting ingredients, so don't give up if the first time you try it doesn't quite work.

EGG

If you're egg-free, you can use one of these replacements in baking and cooking (all the sweet snack and pudding recipes in this book are egg free, though).

- **Aquafaba** (liquid from a can of chickpeas) - Separate the chickpeas, put the liquid in a bowl and whip it with a whisk until it's foamy and forms stiff peaks. 3 tablespoons = 1 egg. You can now also buy this in cartons in the fridge section of supermarkets.

- **Chia or flaxseed egg** - Simply add 1 tablespoon chia or flaxseeds to a bowl and cover with 2½ tablespoons water. Stir and leave for 15 minutes until thick and a gel-like consistency. I find these work best in pancakes, muffins and biscuits.

- **Mashed banana** - Half a ripe mashed banana can be an effective substitute in sweet bakes like muffins.

- **Apple purée** - This works in the same way as banana but has a less distinctive taste. Make your own unsweetened version by adding 500g (1lb 2oz) chopped dessert apples (Braeburn or Gala) into a pan with 120ml (4fl oz) boiling water, then cook, covered, for 20 minutes. Blend. Approx. 50g (1¾oz) apple purée = 1 egg.

- **Egg replacer products** - There are a few available, and they can be useful both for bakes and if you want to make scrambled egg or omelette recipes.

GLUTEN

There's such a wide range of gluten-free ingredients available now, from pasta and bread to flour, oats and breakfast cereals, even beer! So you should be able to find GF substitutes quite easily in the free-from aisle of larger supermarkets. If you're avoiding gluten due to coeliac disease, look for the certified gluten-free stamp on products.

WHEAT

It may be that you are wheat free but not gluten free – in which case choose wheat alternative products and always check packs to ensure wheat is not marked in bold.

NUT BUTTER

If you can tolerate sesame, try tahini in place of nut butter. Other alternatives are seed butters (e.g. pumpkin seed butter), which are really nutritious and often overlooked. There are also soya-based butters available from health food shops which are nut free.

COCONUT

For a substitute for canned coconut milk, I find that using an equal amount of stock with 2–3 tablespoons of Greek-style yoghurt alternative stirred in, plus some ground almonds for sweetness (if nuts are tolerated) works well.

OATS

Quinoa flakes, available in health food shops and some online supermarkets, are an effective oat- and gluten-free substitute which will work in bakes like my Berry & Chia Seed Cookies (see page 175), as well as porridge.

BANANA

Replace mashed banana in recipes with an equal weight of unsweetened apple purée (see previous page).

SOY SAUCE

Try coconut aminos, made from the sap of the coconut plant; it's a dark liquid and handy alternative if you're soya free as the taste is fairly similar. It's also much lower in salt than soy sauce, but it does contain sugar, so be mindful of this if adding it into meals.

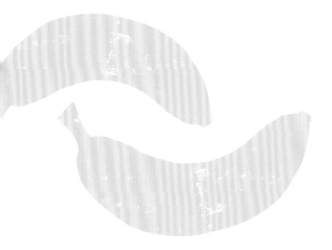

'ACCIDENTALLY' DAIRY-FREE PRODUCTS

Some of my most popular videos on Instagram are where I show products that I spot in supermarkets that you might not expect to be dairy free. It's not a quick process checking labels of everything just in case, but you'll be amazed how many things you'll find. Biscuits, cakes, sauces, garlic bread, coleslaw – the list goes on! One tip is to look for the lower cost/value items as they are more likely to be made with margarine than butter.

Right – on with the fun part! Here are 65 dairy-free recipes that you can enjoy as a family. As well as being delicious, they're all simple, easy to make and have been given the thumbs up from dietitian Lucy.

They're suitable from six months old, unless otherwise stated, and look out for notes of how to adapt for weaning. No salt is added to the recipes, to make them suitable for children, but I do personally choose to season the adults' portions before serving.

An approximate prep and cooking time is included, as well as instructions for keeping in the fridge or freezer if the recipe is suitable for storage.

KEY TO ALLERGENS AND DIETARY REQUIREMENTS

EF = Egg free
GF = Gluten free
NF = Tree nut free (almonds, Brazil nuts, cashews, hazelnuts, walnuts, pecans, pistachios, macadamia nuts)
PF = Peanut free
SF = Soya free
V = Vegetarian
VG = Vegan
WF = Wheat free

Where the recipes contain allergens, make sure you've followed the advice on introducing these first before trying the recipe with your little ones.

If the ingredient is marked with a * it's easily adaptable by using a product free from the relevant allergen, e.g. gluten-free flour/oats, milk/soya-free stock or cheese alternative.

Happy cooking and don't forget to tag me @thedairyfreemum in your creations!

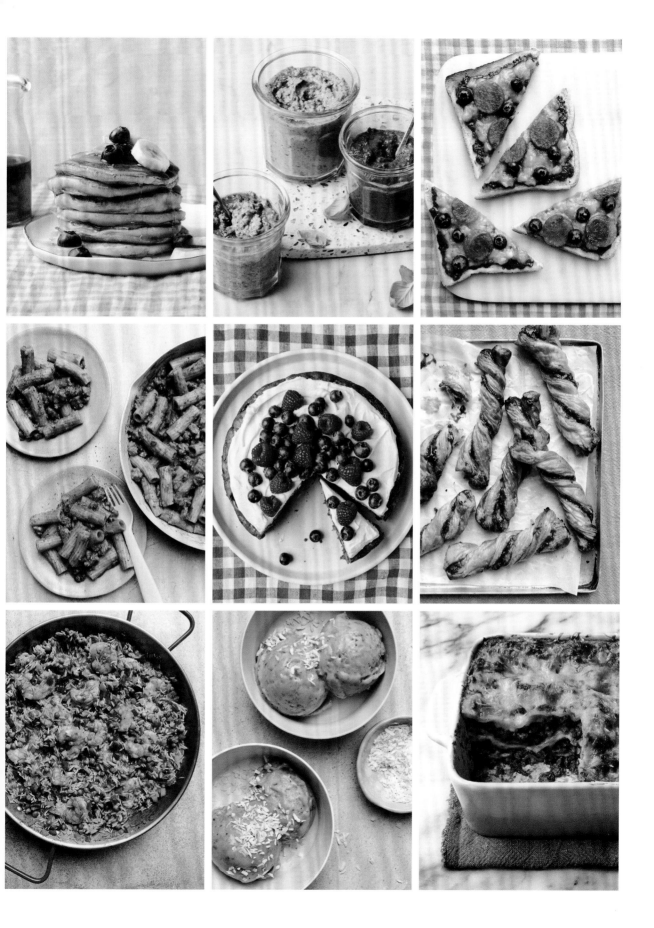

Breakfast

I've always seen breakfast as an ideal opportunity to get some added nutrients in first thing, so I love including natural calcium and iron sources where possible. Setting your family up for the day with a healthy meal feels great - but it also has to be tasty!

There's nothing wrong with a simple brekkie of cereal on busy days (try to choose ones fortified with calcium and iron) and plant-based milk alternative, but I do encourage variety when you have more time to plan.

These recipes are a mix of quick and easy options, alongside some for a more leisurely weekend treat.

Berry Smoothie Bowl

This is my go-to when the kids are ill or teething. It's normal for their appetites to reduce, but as a parent you want to know that some goodness is getting into them! Serve in a bowl with a spoon for littles, or as a drink for older children and adults.

EF, GF*, PF*, SF*, V, VG, WF*

Serves: 1 adult and 2 children

Prep: 5 minutes

2 bananas

2 handfuls of frozen berries

6 tbsp plain yoghurt alternative*

2 tbsp nut butter*

1 tbsp chia seeds

200ml (7fl oz) plant-based milk alternative*

1. Add all the ingredients to a blender and whizz for a minute, then serve.

STORAGE
Keep covered in the fridge for up to 2 days.

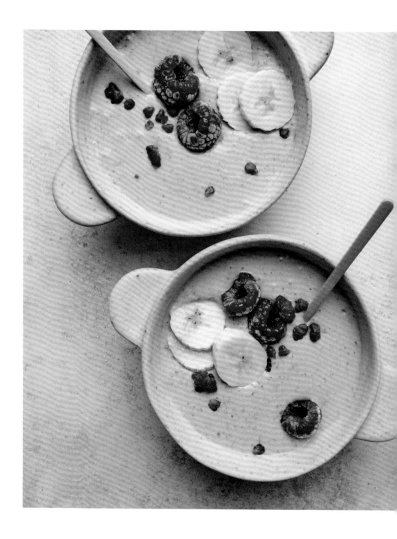

You can also add this to lolly moulds and freeze for homemade smoothie ice pops.

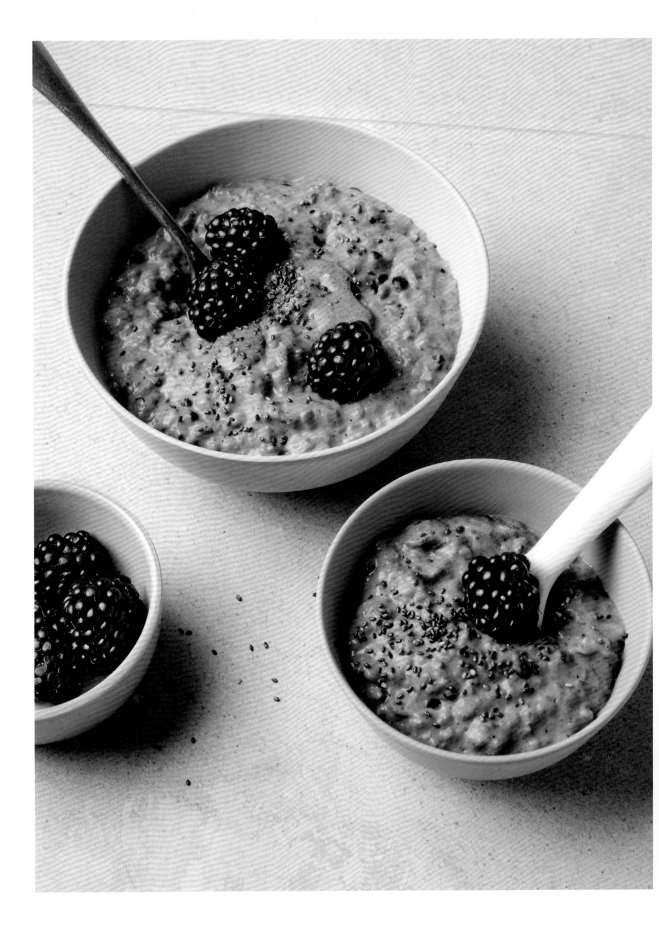

Purple Power Porridge

Kids will love the enticing colour of this porridge, and it's packed with nutrients including calcium, iron and vitamin C. It's also super quick to make and totally delicious. Win, win, win!

EF, GF*, PF, SF*, V, VG, WF*

Serves: 1 adult and 1 child

Prep: 3 minutes, Cook: 7 minutes

60g (2¼oz) porridge oats*

350ml (12fl oz) plant-based milk alternative*, plus extra if needed

100g (3½oz) fresh or frozen blackberries (approx. 2 handfuls)

2 tsp chia seeds

2 tsp almond butter

1. Put the oats and milk alternative in a saucepan on a medium heat.

2. Stir well, bring to the boil, then reduce the heat to low and simmer for 3-4 minutes, stirring regularly.

3. Roughly chop the blackberries and add to the pan, along with the chia seeds. Stir and cook for another 2-3 minutes until the oats are cooked.

4. Take off the heat, stir through the almond butter and add a splash more milk to loosen if needed. Serve once cooled.

STORAGE
Keep covered in the fridge for up to 2 days, reheat and add more milk as needed.

If you can tolerate 'may contain', you can use ready oats which are fortified with extra vitamins and minerals like iron and calcium.

Fluffy Pancakes

Stacks of homemade pancakes have become a weekend breakfast tradition in our house. One of my most popular recipes ever, these are so allergy friendly, also working really well with gluten-free flour. I always make a big batch and freeze what's left, then microwave to defrost when needed, but cut the recipe in half if you'd prefer a smaller amount.

EF, GF*, NF, PF, SF*, V, VG, WF*

Makes: 24

Prep: 10 minutes, Cook: 10 minutes

250g (9oz) self-raising flour*

2 tsp baking powder*

350ml (12fl oz) plant-based milk alternative*

2 tsp vanilla extract

2 tsp maple syrup (omit for under 1s)

oil or butter alternative*, for frying

1. Sift the flour and baking powder into a large bowl.

2. Add the milk alternative, vanilla and maple syrup and whisk well for a couple of minutes until combined with no lumps.

3. Put a large, non-stick frying pan on a low–medium heat and add ½ teaspoon of oil or butter alternative. When melted, stir around the pan until it's evenly coated.

4. Add 1 tablespoon of batter per pancake, then flip when bubbles appear (around 2 minutes) and cook for a further minute. Set aside to cool.

5. Continue with the remaining batter, adding a little more oil or butter alternative if the pan looks dry.

STORAGE
Keep covered in the fridge for up to 1 day.

Freeze in batches between layers of baking paper, defrost in the fridge overnight or use your microwave defrost setting for 30 seconds at a time until fully defrosted. Ensure they're sufficiently cooled before serving.

*For weaning, cut into finger-length strips (just leave out the maple syrup).
Try serving with fresh fruit, plant-based yoghurt alternative and desiccated coconut 'sprinkles'.*

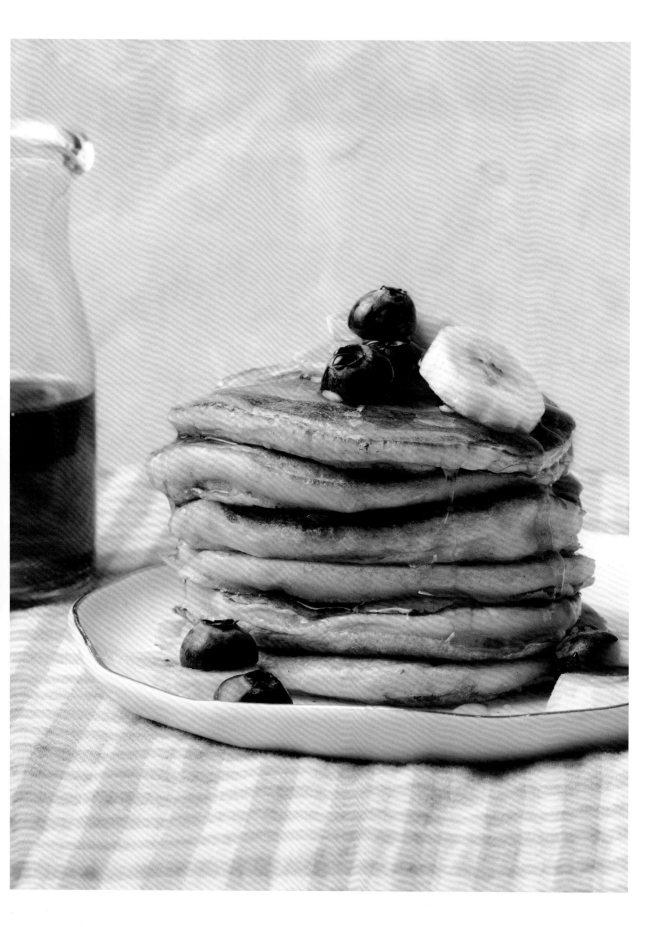

Toast Toppings

You can't go wrong with toast for breakfast, but it's easy to get stuck in a rut with toppings. Here are three tasty ideas which will go down a treat. Slice into wide fingers for weaning.

SUPER-GREEN AVOCADO DIP

EF, GF, NF, PF, SF*, V, VG, WF

If you're an avo-toast fan, you'll love this fresh and nutritious twist. This also makes an incredible pasta sauce!

Serves: 1 adult and 1 child

Prep: 5 minutes

1 ripe avocado

1 handful of spinach leaves, washed

10 basil leaves

juice of ½ lemon

3 tbsp plain yoghurt alternative*

1. Blend all the ingredients together in a blender or food processor and serve.

STORAGE
Keep covered in the fridge for up to 3 days.

Freeze for up to 1 month.

STRAWBERRY CHIA JAM

EF, GF, NF, PF, SF, V, VG, WF

A low sugar alternative to shop-bought jam that's easy to make. Also delicious stirred into porridge, yoghurt alternative or used in my PBJ twists (see page 168).

Makes: 1 jam jar's worth

Prep: 2 minutes, Cook: 8 minutes

250g (9oz) strawberries

1 tbsp maple syrup (omit for under 1s)

2 tbsp chia seeds

1. Remove and discard the green stalks from the strawberries. Cut the berries in half and place in a saucepan with 3 tablespoons of cold water.

2. Cook on a medium heat for 6 minutes, squashing the strawberries down with a masher or wooden spoon until all mashed.

3. Add the maple syrup and chia seeds, stir well, and continue to cook for 2–3 minutes until the consistency looks like jam.

4. Take off the heat (it will continue to thicken as it cools). Serve cold.

STORAGE
Keep in a jam jar or lidded container in the fridge for up to 5 days.

ALMOND BUTTER & RASPBERRY SMASH

EF, GF, PF, SF, V, VG, WF

This tastes like a real treat but is ready in 2 minutes flat – perfect for busy mornings.

Serves: 1

Prep: 2 minutes

1 tbsp smooth almond butter

4 raspberries

1. Add the almond butter to a small bowl and squish the raspberries in.

2. Mix until combined and serve.

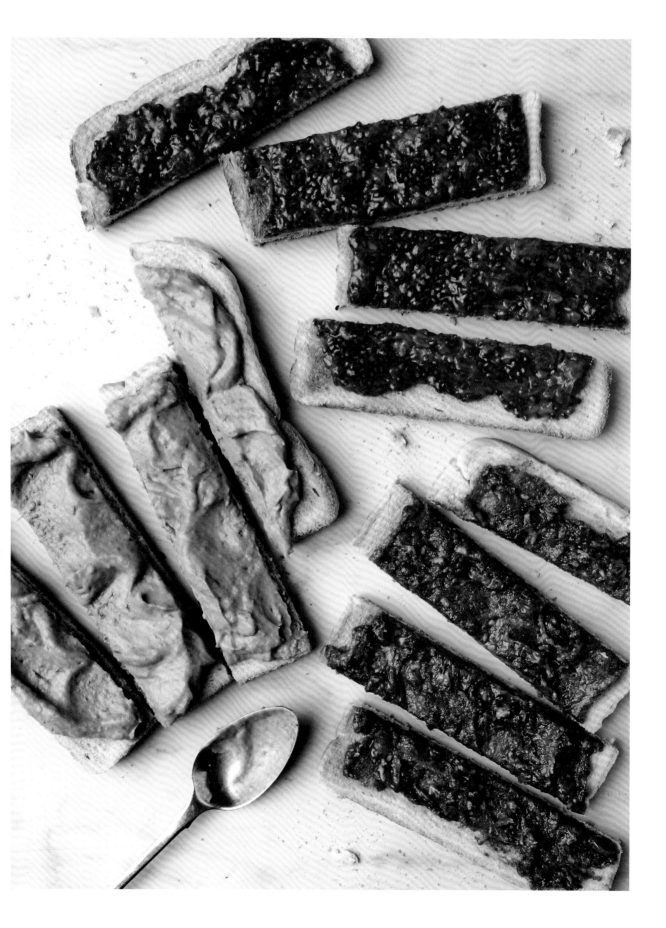

Spiced Nectarine
Overnight Oats

If, like me, you're not a morning person, then prepping breakfast the night before is the ultimate life hack! Five minutes in the evening is all it takes to have this waiting for you the next day. The juicy nectarine and warming cinnamon spice are a match made in heaven.

EF, GF*, NF, PF, SF*, V, VG, WF*

Serves: 1 adult and 2 children

Prep: 5 minutes, Chill: 2+ hours

1 ripe nectarine (or peach)

100g (3½oz) porridge oats*

200ml (7fl oz) plant-based milk alternative*, plus extra to loosen if needed

½ tsp ground cinnamon

1 tsp chia or flax seeds

1. Dice the nectarine flesh finely, discarding the stone.

2. Add to a bowl with the remaining ingredients and mix well.

3. Cover the bowl and pop in the fridge overnight (or for at least 2 hours).

4. When serving, add a dash of milk alternative to loosen if required.

STORAGE
Keep covered in the fridge for up to 2 days.

Any soft, ripe fruit will work well here. You can also heat this on the hob or in the microwave if you prefer your oats warmed.

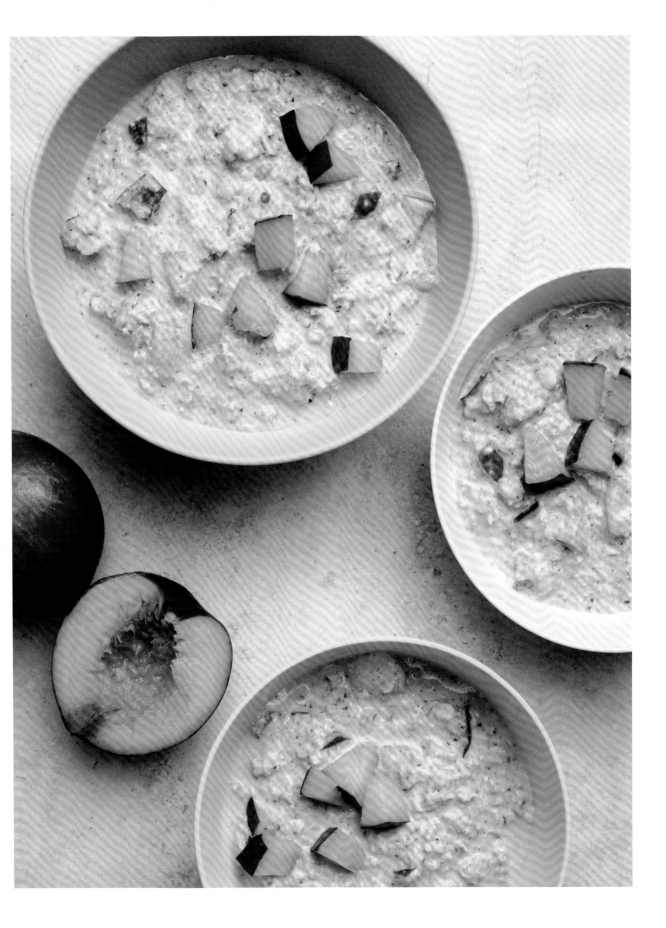

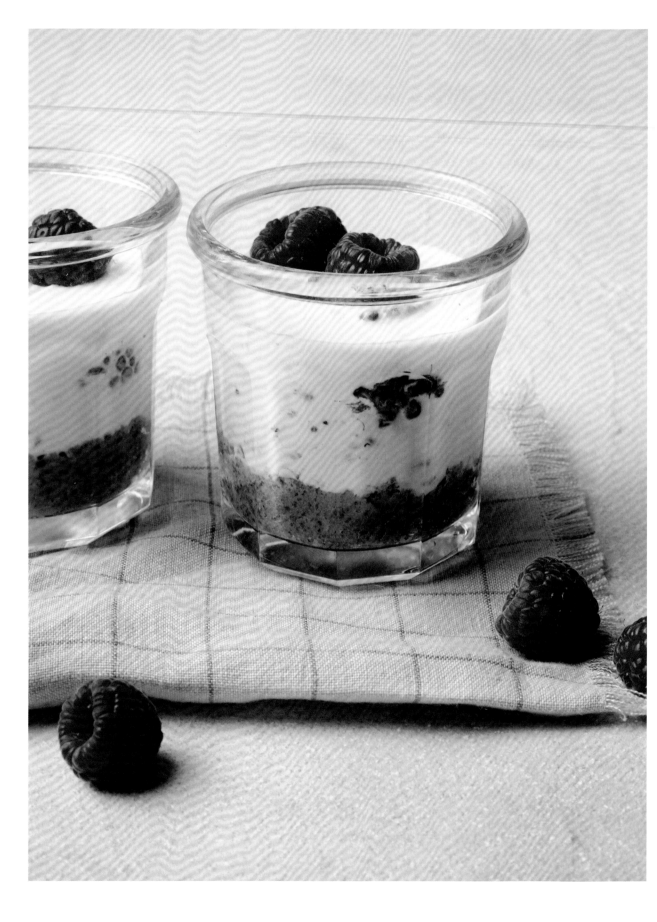

Overnight Raspberry 'Cheesecake'

You may have seen these clever wheat biscuit cheesecakes doing the rounds on social media after going viral. They're a doddle to make, and a great way of serving iron-rich breakfast cereal in a more interesting way.

EF, NF, PF, SF*, V, VG

Serves: 1 adult or 2 children

Prep: 5 minutes, Chill: 2+ hours

---

2 wheat biscuits

125ml (4fl oz) plant-based milk alternative*

150g (5½oz) Greek-style yoghurt alternative*

30g (1oz) raspberries

1. Break the wheat biscuits into a small dish or container.

2. Add the milk alternative and leave to soak for 1 minute, then mix well and press down firmly with a spoon so it's compacted into the dish.

3. Spread over the Greek-style yoghurt alternative, then break up the raspberries on top and swirl in.

4. Cover and chill in the fridge overnight (or for at least 2 hours).

STORAGE
Keep covered in the fridge for up to 1 day.

Experiment with mixing different toppings into the yoghurt, e.g. sliced banana, peanut butter or even crushed dairy-free biscuits as a treat for older kids and adults.

Egg-Free French Toast

Crispy French toast with a lovely custardy centre and natural sweetness from the banana, without the egg. The trick here is to use stale bread, so leave it out overnight, if possible, to achieve that desired crunch on the outside. If you forget, lightly toast and cool the bread before starting.

EF, GF*, NF, PF, SF*, V, VG, WF*

Serves: 1 adult and 1 child

Prep: 6 minutes, Cook: 6 minutes

1 tbsp plain flour*

100ml (3½fl oz) plant-based milk alternative*

½ ripe banana

¼ tsp ground cinnamon

1 tsp butter alternative* or margarine*

2 slices of stale bread*

1. Mix the flour and milk alternative in a shallow bowl, then whisk well for a couple of minutes until combined.

2. Mash the banana and add to the milk mixture, along with the cinnamon, and stir to combine.

3. Heat the butter alternative or margarine in a non-stick frying pan on a low-medium heat until melted and starting to bubble.

4. Dunk the bread into the milk mix on both sides, then add to the pan.

5. Cook for 3 minutes on each side until golden. Cut into halves and serve.

For weaning, cut into thick strips that can be held in the fist.
Serve with Greek-style yoghurt alternative and fruit or drizzle the adult's portion with maple syrup.

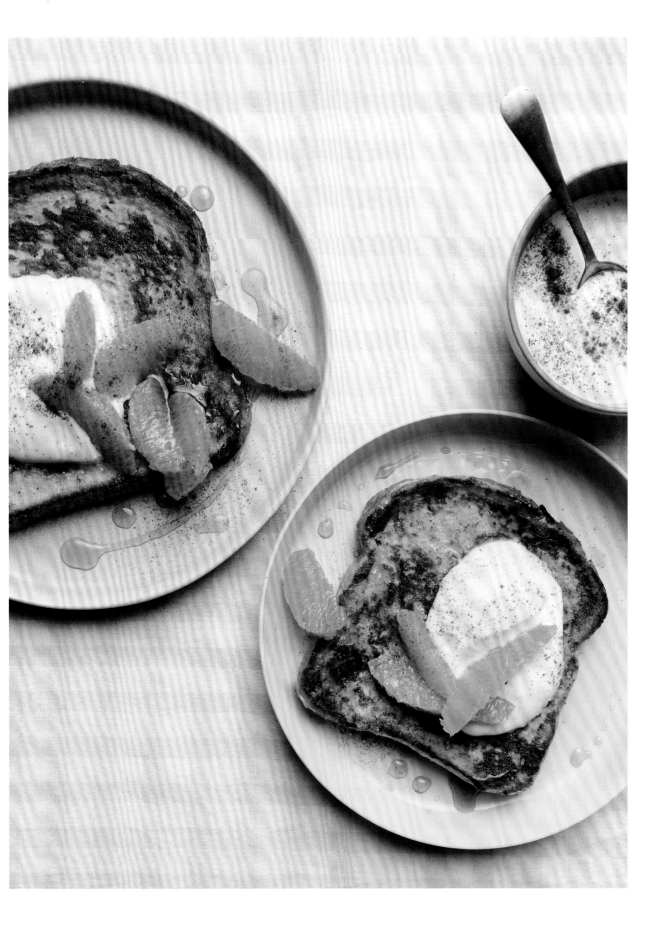

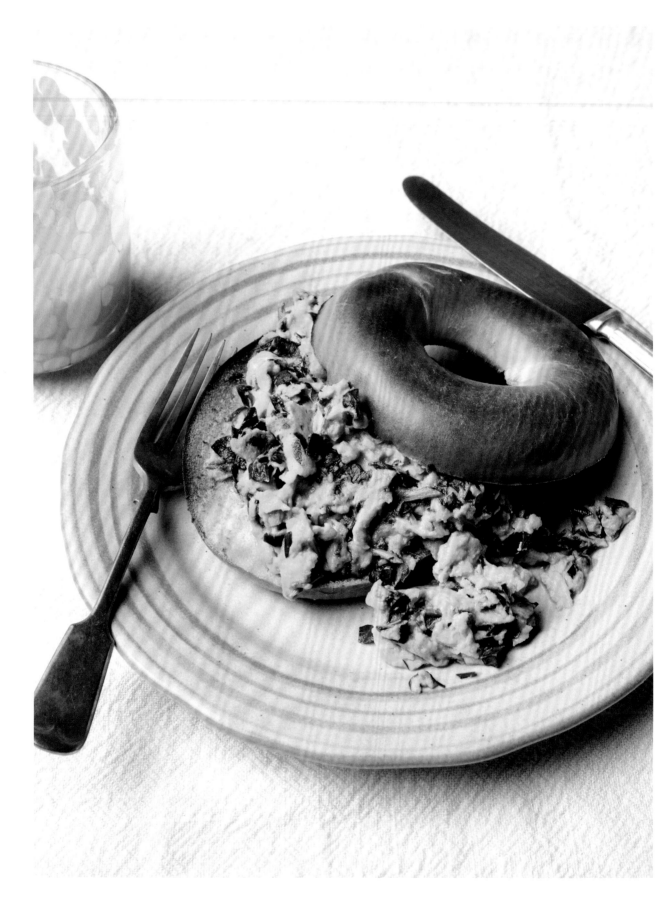

Nutrient-Boost Scrambled Eggs

Perfectly fluffy eggs are combined with iron-rich spinach and nutritional yeast for a savoury punch. These also make a great lunch option.

GF*, NF, PF, SF*, V, WF*

Serves: 1 adult or 2 children

Prep: 6 minutes, Cook: 3 minutes

1 handful of spinach leaves

2 tbsp plant-based milk alternative*

2 tbsp nutritional yeast

2 large eggs

½ tbsp olive oil

Toast, bagel or tortilla wrap*, to serve

1. Wash and finely chop the spinach, then add to a bowl with the milk alternative and nutritional yeast.

2. Beat the eggs and add to the bowl, then stir to combine.

3. Heat the oil in a non-stick frying pan on a low heat.

4. Add the egg mix and cook slowly, stirring often, for 2–3 minutes until cooked through.

5. Serve with toast, a bagel or even a tortilla wrap to make a breakfast burrito.

If you're egg free, try this recipe using one of the plant-based egg replacer products available, which are suitable for scrambling.

Banana Peanut Butter Bites

Everyone will love these for a fun family breakfast - they taste as good as they look!

EF, GF*, NF, SF*, V, VG, WF*

Serves: 1 adult or 2 children

Prep: 6 minutes, Cook: 4 minutes

25ml (1fl oz) plant-based milk alternative*

2 slices of bread*

1 tbsp smooth peanut butter

2 small bananas, peeled

1 tbsp butter alternative*

1. Pour the milk alternative into a shallow bowl.

2. Remove the crusts from the bread and flatten the slices completely with a rolling pin.

3. Spread the peanut butter over the bread.

4. Place a banana on top of each slice of bread and roll up tightly into a sausage shape. Dunk the bread roll-ups in the milk alternative so they are completely covered.

5. In a large non-stick frying pan, melt the butter alternative on a medium heat. When starting to bubble, place the roll-ups seam-side down for 1 minute, then cook, turning regularly, until golden all over (this should take 3-4 minutes in total).

6. Remove from the pan, cool slightly and cut each roll into bite-sized pieces.

Peanut butter can be replaced with another nut butter, jam or chocolate spread.

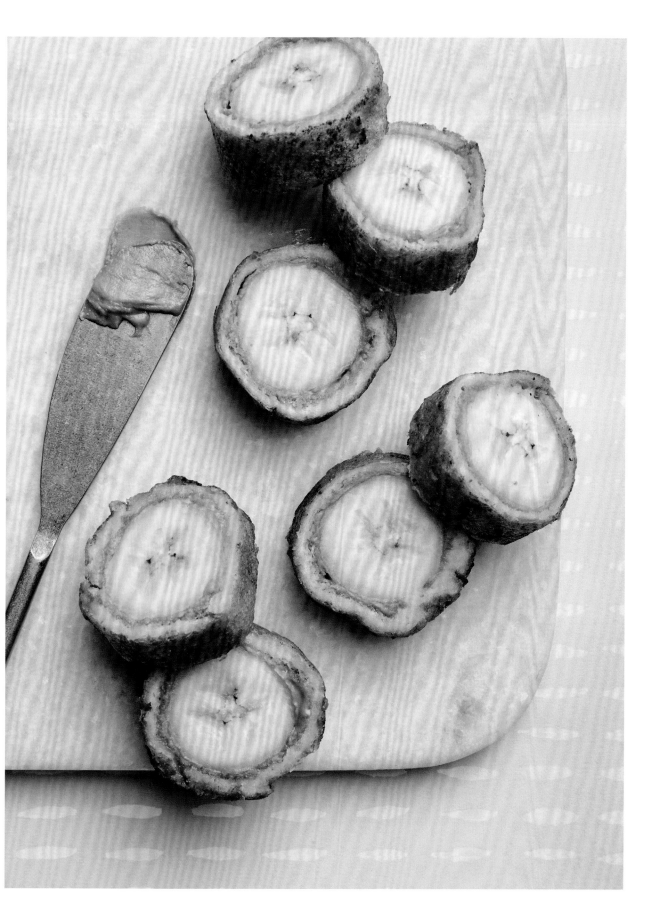

Lunch

I'm often told that you find lunch the trickiest meal to think of ideas for, so here are lots of tasty options. In my mind, lunch should always be quick and easy to prepare, so most of these recipes are ready in 15 minutes or less.

Avocado Cheeze Roll-Ups

Creamy avocado pairs so well with melted cheeze in this fun twist on a toastie. The trick to a great roll-up is to make sure the bread is completely flattened, then take care not to overfill it. These are a great size for baby to hold when weaning.

EF, GF*, NF, PF, SF*, V, VG, WF*

Serves: 1 adult or 2 children

Prep: 6 minutes, Cook: 4 minutes

½ ripe avocado

15g (½oz) Cheddar alternative*

1 tsp butter alternative* or margarine*

2 slices of bread*

1. Mash the avocado with a fork. Finely grate the Cheddar alternative. Melt the butter alternative or margarine.

2. Remove crusts from the bread, then flatten the slices with a rolling pin.

3. Spread the mashed avocado over the bread, then sprinkle over the Cheddar alternative.

4. Put a dry, non-stick frying pan on a low heat.

5. Make the roll-ups by rolling the bread tightly along the longest edge to form a cylinder shape. Brush all over with the melted butter alternative or margarine.

6. Add the roll-ups, seam-side down, to the frying pan. Cook gently for 1-2 minutes turning regularly, until golden all over.

7. Remove from the heat and slice each roll-up in half.

STORAGE
Best eaten fresh.

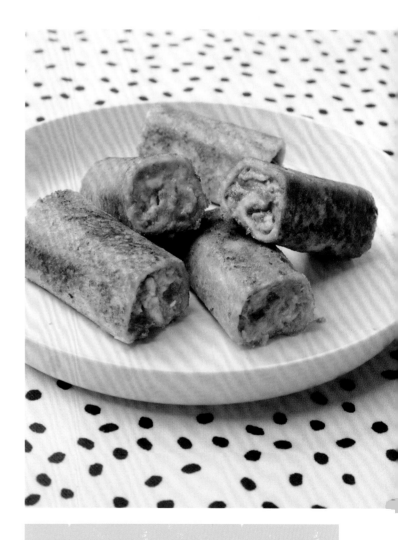

Try other fillings with the cheeze – like ham, pesto or tuna. Save the crusts for Bread Crust 'Churros' (see page 185)!

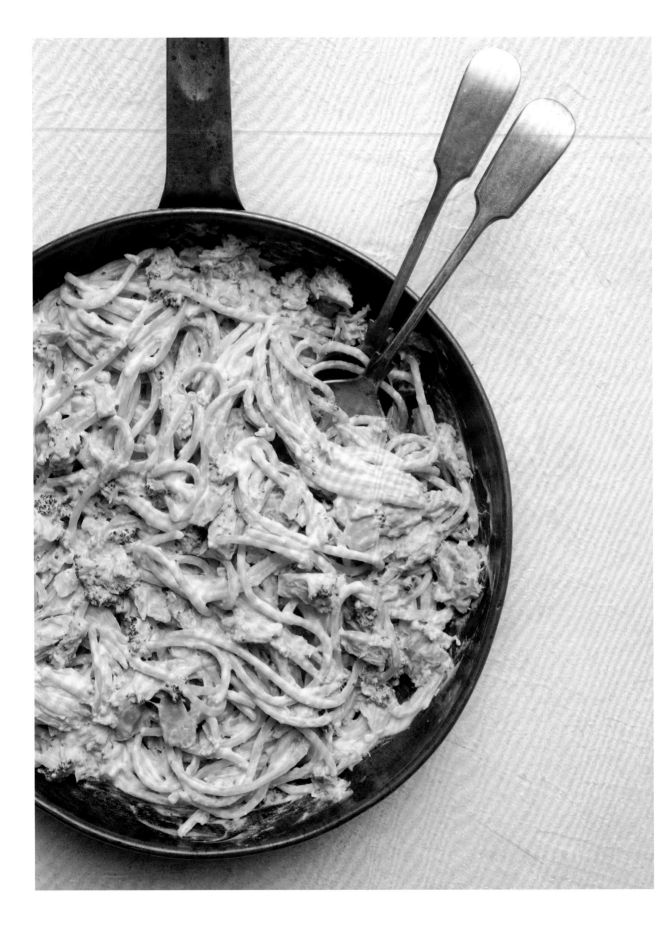

Creamy Tuna & Broccoli Spaghetti

A simple and tasty pasta dish that's deceptively nutrient-rich, with good sources of protein, iodine, calcium and vitamin C. Use quick-cook spaghetti if you want to speed this up further.

EF, GF*, NF, PF, SF*, WF*

Serves: 1 adult and 1 child

Prep: 3 minutes, Cook: 12 minutes

100g (3½oz) broccoli

150g (5½oz) spaghetti*

oil, for cooking

1 tsp garlic paste

4 tbsp soft cheese alternative*

145g (5oz) can tuna chunks (in spring water)

juice of ¼ lemon

1 tbsp nutritional yeast (optional)

1. Chop the broccoli into florets, discarding any of the long stalks.

2. Put a large saucepan of water on to boil, then add the spaghetti. For the last 5 minutes of cooking time, add the broccoli florets.

3. Reserve a cup of the starchy pasta water, then drain the pasta and broccoli.

4. Return the empty pan to the hob, then add a splash of oil and the garlic paste and cook on a low heat, stirring, for 1 minute.

5. Add the soft cheese alternative, along with 3 tablespoons of the reserved pasta water, stirring until melted and combined.

6. Drain the tuna and add to the pan, along with the lemon juice and nutritional yeast.

7. Chop the broccoli florets into small pieces and add to the pan with the drained spaghetti, mix well until all coated, then serve.

STORAGE
Keep covered in the fridge for up to 2 days. If reheating, add a splash of water to loosen if needed.

Not suitable for freezing.

For weaning, this can be puréed, or consider replacing the spaghetti with rigatoni or fusilli for baby to be able to hold. Baby pasta or orzo is also a great option when transitioning with textures.
If reheating, add a splash of water if needed to loosen.

Mexican Bean Quesadilla

Quesadillas are such a great option to rustle up for lunch. Pack in some plant-based protein with these mildly spiced, flavourful toasted wraps which will be loved by kids and adults alike.

EF, GF*, NF, PF, SF*, V, VG, WF*

Serves: 1 adult or 2 children

Prep: 5 minutes, Cook: 5 minutes

---

3 cherry or plum tomatoes (or ½ salad tomato)

60g (2¼oz) black beans (drained weight)

1 tbsp cooked sweetcorn

¼ tsp ground cumin

¼ tsp ground coriander

20g (¾oz) Cheddar alternative*, finely grated

1 tortilla wrap* (or 2 mini wraps)

1 tbsp plain yoghurt alternative*

1. Dice the tomatoes finely.

2. Rinse the beans, place in a bowl, then mash roughly with a fork.

3. Add the sweetcorn, cumin, coriander, tomatoes, grated Cheddar alternative and yoghurt alternative. Mix well.

4. Spread the mix evenly over half the wrap, then fold the wrap over to make a crescent shape.

5. Heat a dry frying pan on a low heat, then add the folded wrap and cook for 2-3 minutes on each side until lightly golden.

6. Cool, slice and serve.

STORAGE
Best eaten fresh.

Any canned beans can be used, or if you're legume-free, swap for chopped cooked chicken or cubes of cooked sweet potato.

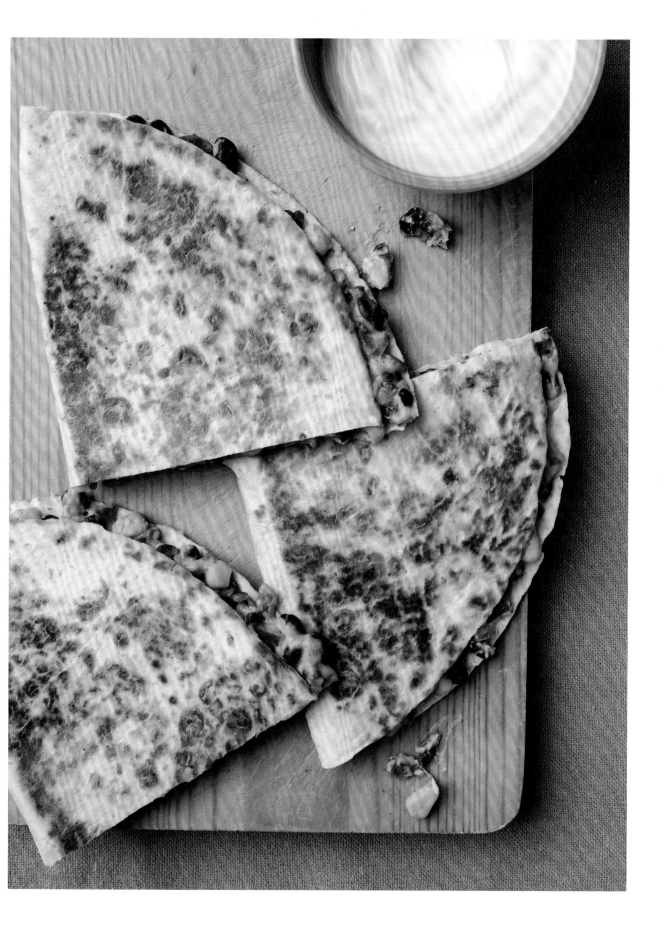

Pesto Three Ways

Pesto is a handy staple to have in the fridge, but most shop-bought options contain milk, soya and/or have added salt. Here are three options which are all delicious when stirred through pasta or rice, in toasties or even when used as a pizza base.

PEA

EF, GF, NF, PF, SF, V, VG, WF

One of my most popular recipes – super fresh and tasty!

Makes: 1 small jar

Prep: 5 minutes, Cook: 4 minutes

125g (4½oz) frozen peas

15g (½oz) basil leaves

1 garlic clove, peeled

100ml (3½fl oz) olive oil

2 tbsp nutritional yeast

juice of ½ lemon

1. Cook the peas in a pan of boiling water for 4 minutes, then drain and cool.

2. Add to a food processor with all the remaining ingredients and blend.

ROASTED RED PEPPER

EF, GF*, NF, PF, SF*, V, VG, WF*

Roasting the red peppers gives a sweetness, while breadcrumbs act as a nut substitute for a classic pesto texture.

Makes: 1 small jar

Prep: 10 minutes, Cook: 25 minutes

2 red (bell) peppers

3 tbsp olive oil, plus extra to loosen if needed

15g (½oz) basil leaves

1 garlic clove, peeled

2 tbsp panko breadcrumbs* (or gluten-free breadcrumbs)

2 tbsp nutritional yeast

1. Preheat the oven to 220°C/ Fan 200°C/425°F/Gas Mark 7.

2. Chop the peppers into large 5cm (2in) chunks, coat in 1 tablespoon of the olive oil, then place on a baking tray, skin-side down.

3. Roast in the oven for 25 minutes until the edges are charring.

4. Cool the peppers, then add to a food processor with the remaining olive oil, the basil, garlic, breadcrumbs and nutritional yeast, and blend until smooth. If the pesto looks too thick, add another tablespoon of olive oil and blend again.

BASIL & CASHEW

EF, GF, PF, SF, V, VG, WF

A creamy, nutty version that's rich in protein and healthy fats.

Makes: 1 small jar

Prep: 35 minutes

75g (2½oz) plain unsalted cashews

30g (1oz) basil leaves

1 garlic clove, peeled

100ml (3½fl oz) olive oil

1½ tbsp nutritional yeast

juice of ½ lemon

1. Soak the cashews in a bowl of just-boiled water for 30 minutes (this makes them much easier to blend), then drain and discard the water.

2. Add the cashews to a food processor with all the remaining ingredients and blend.

STORAGE
All three pestos will keep in the fridge (covered) for up to 4 days, or can be frozen for up to 6 months.

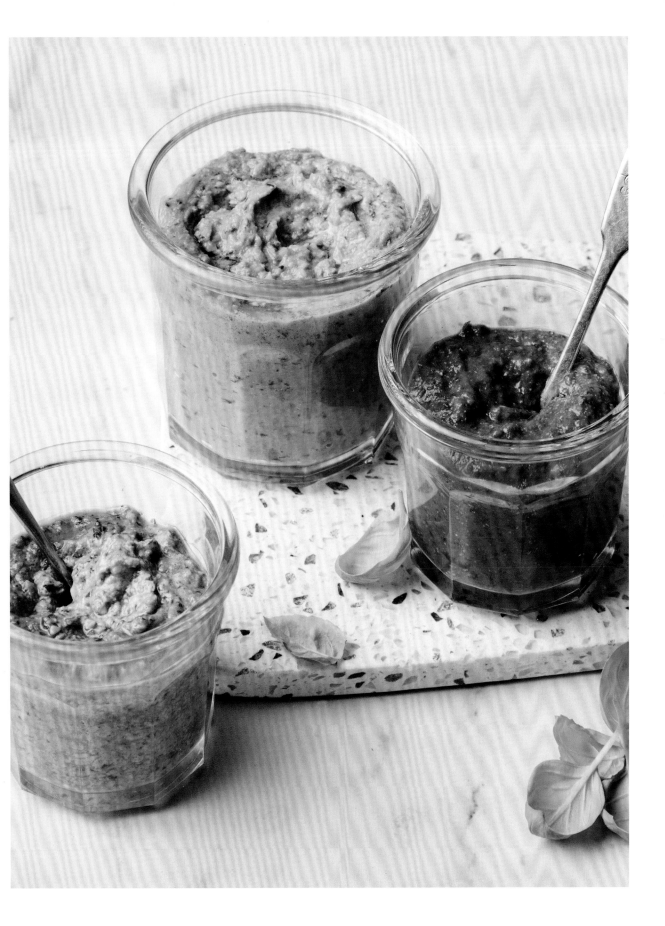

Cheat Chicken Noodle Soup

There are few meals more comforting than a hot bowl of chicken soup, but it can be time intensive to make, plus shop-bought versions are often high in salt. So here's a speedy cheat version that you can have on the table in minutes!

EF*, GF*, NF, PF, SF*, WF*

Serves: 1 adult and 1 child

Prep: 5 minutes, Cook: 10 minutes

1 litre (35fl oz) (low-salt) hot chicken stock*

1 tsp ginger paste

½ tsp garlic paste

1 tsp mild curry powder (optional, for a mild spice)

50g (1¾oz) frozen or canned sweetcorn

1 nest (approx. 60g/2¼oz) fine egg noodles* (or vermicelli rice noodles)

100g (3½oz) cooked chicken breast

1. Add the hot stock to a large saucepan on a medium heat.

2. Bring to the boil, then add the ginger and garlic pastes, plus curry powder if using, then reduce the heat to low.

3. Add the sweetcorn and nest of noodles and cook for 4-5 minutes, stirring often, until the noodles are soft.

4. Meanwhile, chop the cooked chicken into small slices.

5. Ladle the soup into bowls, then top with the chicken.

STORAGE
Keep covered in the fridge for up to 2 days.

Freeze for up to 3 months.

If you have more time, fry some onion, celery and carrot in a little oil for a few minutes before adding the stock for extra flavour. Some chopped fresh herbs scattered on top work a treat too.

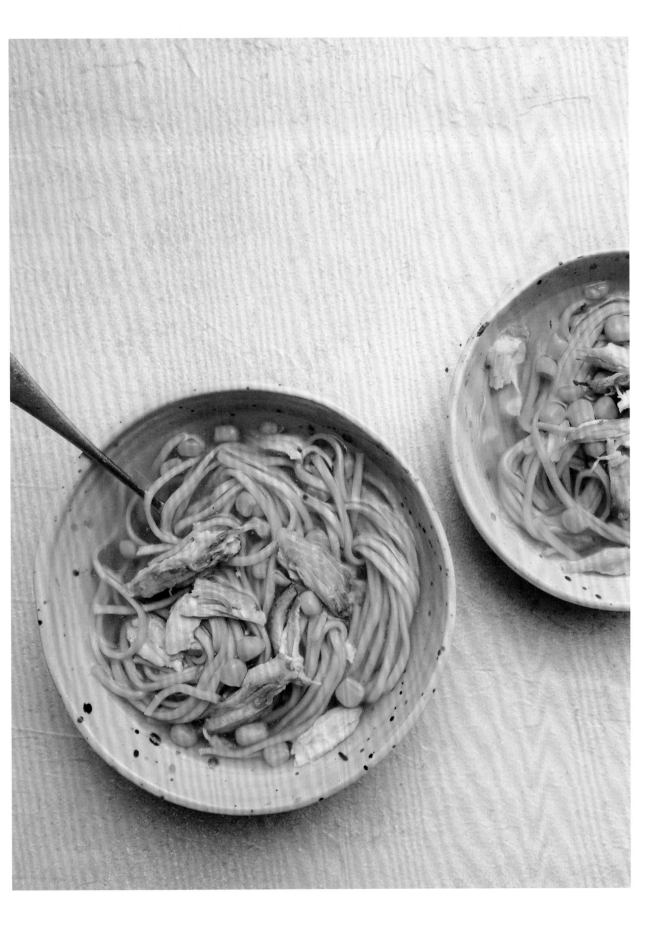

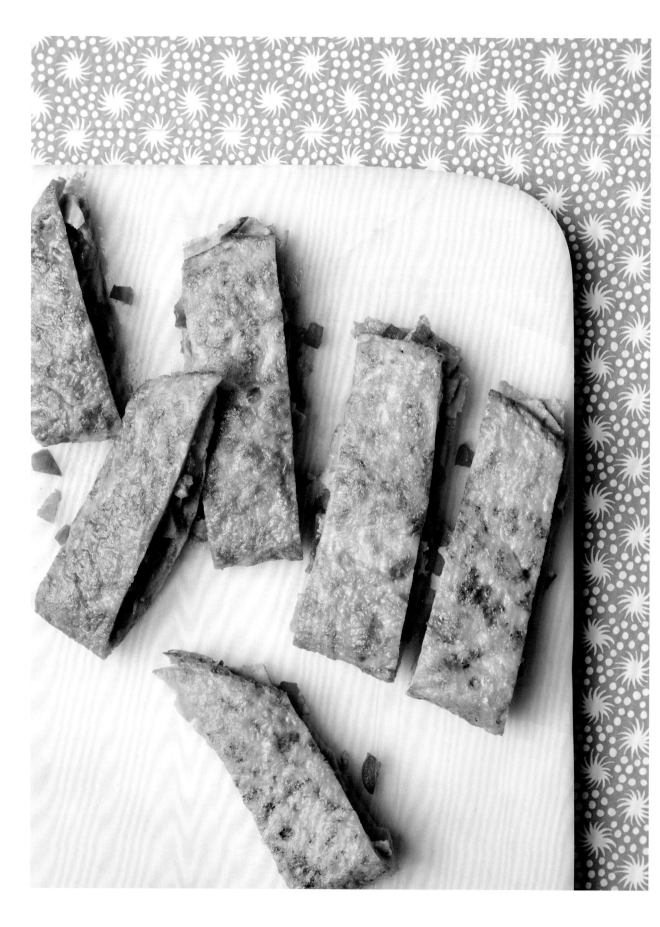

Ham, Pepper & Tomato Omelette

Omelettes are a brilliant way to include iron-rich eggs in your family's diet, and here the delicious pepper and tomato give a vitamin C boost to aid that iron absorption.

GF*, NF, PF, SF, WF*

Serves: 1 adult or 2 children

Prep: 5 minutes, Cook: 10 minutes

½ red (bell) pepper

4 cherry or plum tomatoes

2 slices of ham*

1 tsp oil, for cooking

3 large eggs

1 tbsp nutritional yeast (optional)

1. Dice the pepper and tomatoes finely. Chop the ham into small pieces.

2. Heat the oil in a large, non-stick frying pan over a low–medium heat.

3. Add the pepper and tomatoes and cook for 5 minutes, stirring often, until softened. Remove on to a plate.

4. Beat the eggs in a bowl, then add to the pan, swirling round until evenly spread.

5. Sprinkle over the nutritional yeast (if using) and cook for a few minutes until the eggs are no longer translucent.

6. Add the peppers, tomatoes and ham to one half of the eggs, cook for 1 minute, then using a non-stick spatula, fold the omelette in half to make a crescent shape.

7. Cook for a further minute, remove from the pan, cool and slice.

STORAGE
Keep covered in the fridge for up to 1 day.

Not suitable for freezing.

For weaning, cut the omelette into thick strips that baby can hold.

Sandwich Ideas

Sandwiches are such a classic lunch staple, but if your childhood lunchboxes consisted of cheese and butter sarnies then a) you're not alone and b) you may be seeking dairy-free ideas! Here are four of my favourites; they each use a different bread base (bread, bagel, wrap, toastie) but are all interchangeable, so feel free to mix them up.

CREAMY TUNA & SWEETCORN SANDWICH

EF, GF*, NF, PF, SF*, WF*

Substituting the traditional mayonnaise for a yoghurt alternative reduces the salt content but still gives this filling a creamy and satisfying texture.

Serves: 1

Prep: 5 minutes

½ x 145g (5oz) can of tuna chunks (in spring water)

1½ tbsp plain or Greek-style yoghurt alternative*

2 tbsp canned sweetcorn

2 slices of bread*

1 tsp butter alternative* or margarine*

1. Drain the tuna and add to a bowl, then mix in the yoghurt alternative and sweetcorn.

2. Spread one slice of bread with butter alternative or margarine, then top with the tuna mix, and finally the second slice of bread. Slice and serve.

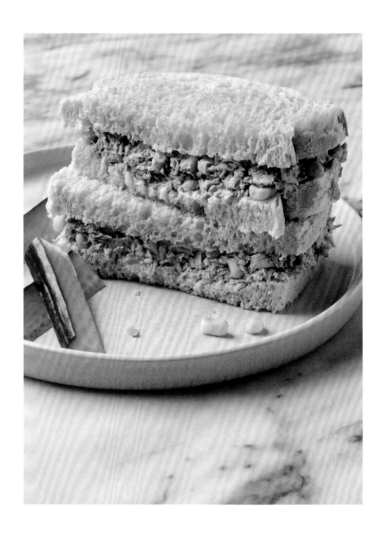

Choose a low-salt ham for babies and younger children.

HAM, SOFT CHEEZE & CUCUMBER BAGEL

EF, GF*, NF, PF, SF*, WF*

Bagels are a great alternative to sandwiches and tend to be dairy free (always check packs!). I like mine lightly toasted before filling.

Serves: 1

Prep: 5 minutes

1 bagel or bagel thin*, halved

2.5cm (1in) piece of cucumber

1 tbsp soft cheese alternative*

2 slices of ham*

1. Lightly toast the bagel, then leave to cool.

2. Meanwhile, cut the cucumber into thin slices.

3. Spread the soft cheese alternative over one half of the bagel, then top with the cucumber slices and finally the ham.

4. Top with the other half of the bagel, slice and serve.

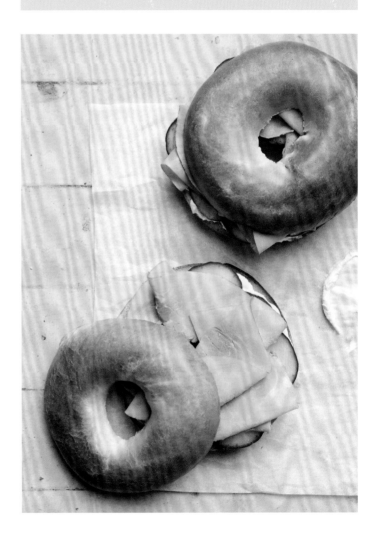

HUMMUS & CARROT WRAP

EF, GF*, NF, PF, SF*, V, VG, WF*

Homemade hummus is really easy to make, and a healthier option than shop-bought, which is usually high in salt. Grated carrot adds a lovely freshness to this simple wrap.

Serves: 1

Prep: 10 minutes

HUMMUS

400g (14oz) can chickpeas

1½ tbsp tahini (sesame paste)

1 small garlic clove, peeled

juice of ½ lemon

2 tbsp olive oil

½ tsp ground cumin

WRAP

1 small carrot

1 tortilla wrap*

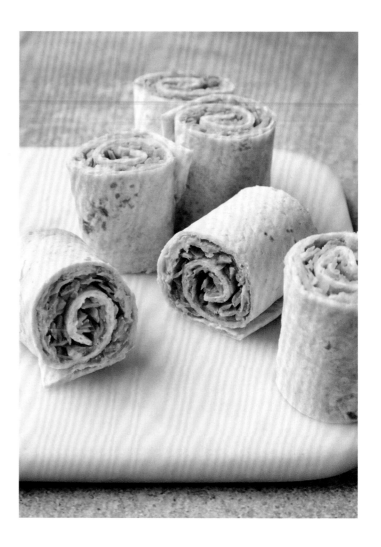

Hummus

1. Drain the chickpeas, reserving the liquid (aquafaba) in a bowl, then rinse.

2. Add the chickpeas and all the remaining ingredients to a blender with 1 tablespoon of aquafaba and blend, adding a tablespoon of aquafaba at a time until it's your desired consistency.

Wrap

1. Peel, then grate your carrot.

2. Spread 2 tablespoons of hummus on the wrap, then top with the grated carrot.

3. Roll up the wrap tightly and serve.

STORAGE

Hummus will keep covered in the fridge for up to 3 days.

Tahini is a paste made from sesame seeds; as this is an allergen make sure you follow guidance for introducing sesame if you haven't offered it before.

If you're egg free, keep the remaining aquafaba for use in baking (see page 76).

APPLE & PEANUT BUTTER TOASTIE

EF, GF*, NF, SF*, V, VG, WF*

There's no reason why sandwiches should all be savoury! This is such a tasty option and also works really well with mashed banana instead of the apple.

Serves: 1

Prep: 5 minutes, Cook: 5 minutes

1 apple

¼ tsp ground cinnamon

1 tbsp smooth peanut butter

2 slices of bread*

butter alternative* or margarine*

1. Peel, core, then grate your apple. Pick up in your hand and squeeze out the excess moisture for a couple of seconds – you don't want it to dry completely though.

2. Add the grated apple to a bowl with the cinnamon and mix.

3. Spread the peanut butter over one slice of bread, then top evenly with the apple mix.

4. Place the other slice of bread on top, then, with a knife, spread the top evenly with butter alternative or margarine.

5. Heat a dry, non-stick frying pan on a low heat.

6. Add the sandwich, butter-side down, then spread the top evenly with butter alternative or margarine.

7. Cook for 2 minutes on each side until golden.

8. Cool, slice and serve.

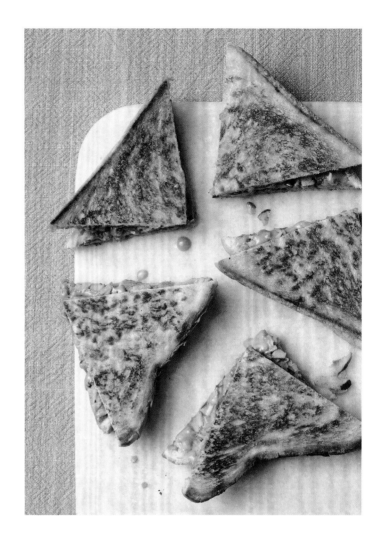

Family Favourites

When dreaming of writing this book, long before it actually became a reality, I knew I wanted to create a section of classic family meals. Ones that lots of you message me about desperately seeking a recipe for, and ones that you might not realise you can make dairy free. These dinners are delicious, comforting and completely embody my 'no one misses out' principle. I hope they become favourites of yours too.

Lasagne

Officially my most requested recipe of all time... no pressure! Well, this one shouldn't disappoint - who could resist those delicious layers and crispy top? It's a total crowd-pleaser and well worth the effort.

EF*, GF*, NF, PF, SF*, WF*

Serves: 4 adults and 2 children

Prep: 1 hour 15 minutes, Cook: 40 minutes

FOR THE MEAT SAUCE

1 onion

1 celery stick

½ courgette

2 garlic cloves, peeled

1 large carrot

1 tbsp oil

500g (1lb 2oz) minced beef (or pork)

500ml (18fl oz) tomato passata

200ml (7fl oz) hot (low-salt) beef stock*

1 tbsp tomato purée

1 tbsp dried mixed herbs

FOR THE WHITE SAUCE

90g (3¼oz) butter alternative* or margarine*

65g (2¼oz) plain flour*

600ml (20fl oz) plant-based milk alternative*

3 tbsp nutritional yeast

FOR THE LASAGNE

dried lasagne sheets*

75g (2½oz) Cheddar or mozzarella alternative*

1. Prep your ingredients - dice the onion, celery, courgette and garlic finely. Peel, then grate the carrot.

2. To make your meat sauce, in a large saucepan, heat the oil on a low-medium heat, then cook the onion, celery and carrot for 5 minutes, stirring often. Add the garlic and courgette for a further 2 minutes.

3. Turn up the heat, push the veg to one side of the pan and add the minced beef to the empty side. Cook, stirring, for several minutes until brown all over, then combine with the veg.

4. Add the passata, hot stock, tomato purée and mixed herbs. Bring to the boil, then reduce the heat to low and simmer, uncovered, for 30 minutes until thickened. Cover the pan and leave to cool.

5. Meanwhile, make your white sauce. In a saucepan, melt the butter alternative or margarine on a low-medium heat. When bubbling, add the flour and cook, stirring, for 1 minute. Gradually add the milk alternative, whisking constantly until the liquid is absorbed and repeat until all combined. Finally, add the nutritional yeast and stir well for a further 2 minutes. Cover with a lid and leave to cool.

6. Preheat the oven to 200°C/ Fan 180°C /400°F/Gas Mark 6.

7. Spoon one third of the meat sauce into a large, ovenproof dish and spread evenly. Arrange the lasagne sheets in a single layer over the top, then spoon over a third of the white sauce, again spreading evenly. Repeat these steps, finishing with a layer of the white sauce.

8. Finely grate the cheese alternative and sprinkle evenly over the top.

9. Bake for 35-40 minutes until golden and bubbling.

STORAGE
Keep covered in the fridge for up to 2 days.

Freeze for up to 3 months.

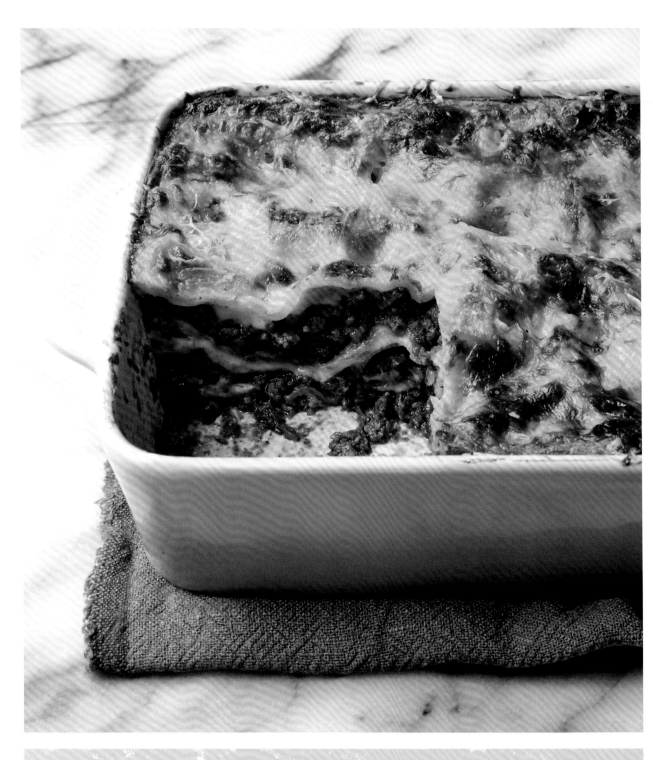

Leaving the sauces to cool before assembling the lasagne helps to keep the layers more separate, but it's not essential if you're tight on time.
You can prepare the lasagne up to a day ahead of time, and keep it covered in the fridge ready to bake.

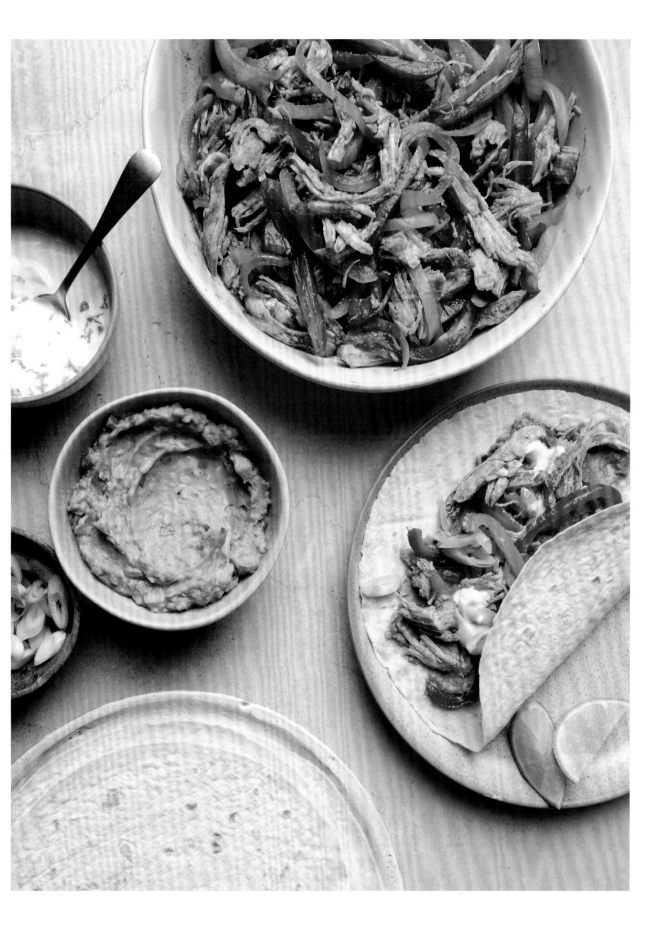

Pulled Chicken Fajitas
with Guacamole & Lime 'Yoghurt'

A flavourful family feast! I find meals like this, which have multiple elements for everyone to choose from, can help encourage even fussy eaters to get excited about dinner. The 'pulling' technique of preparing the chicken makes it so juicy and succulent – much more so than chunks, which have a tendency to dry out.

EF, GF*, NF, PF, SF*, WF*

Serves: 2 adults and 2 children

Prep: 15 minutes, Cook: 30 minutes

FOR THE MAIN DISH

spice mix made from: 1 tsp ground smoked paprika, 1 tsp ground cumin, ½ tsp ground coriander, ½ tsp dried oregano

1 tbsp oil, plus extra for cooking

2 chicken breasts

1 onion

2 (bell) peppers (I use red and yellow)

1 tbsp tomato purée

150ml (5fl oz) hot (low-salt) chicken stock*

6 tortilla wraps*

FOR THE GUACAMOLE

1 ripe avocado

1 handful of coriander leaves

juice of ½ lime

FOR THE LIME 'YOGHURT'

150g (5½oz) Greek-style yoghurt alternative*

juice of ½ lime

OPTIONAL EXTRA TOPPINGS

sliced spring onions

grated cheese alternative*

Serve the fajitas deconstructed for weaning and younger children, as they can still enjoy all the separate components without the messiness of a wrap.

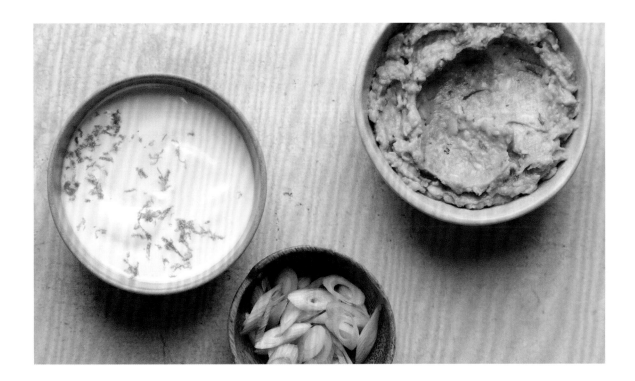

1. Make the spice mix by combining the spices in a bowl, then add 1 tablespoon of oil and mix well. Use this to coat the chicken breasts all over, then set aside to marinate.

2. Slice the onion and peppers into thin strips.

3. Add the tomato purée to your hot chicken stock and mix well.

4. In a wide non-stick lidded saucepan, heat 1 teaspoon of oil on a medium–high heat. Add the onion and pepper slices and cook, stirring often, for 3 minutes. Remove from the pan into a bowl.

5. Keep the pan on the heat and add the marinated chicken breasts. Cook for 2½ minutes on each side.

6. Add the tomato stock mix, bring to the boil, then reduce the heat to low, cover the pan with its lid and simmer for 12 minutes.

7. Meanwhile, make your guacamole. Mash the avocado flesh in a bowl until smooth. Finely chop the coriander and add to the avocado, along with the lime juice, and mix well. Also prepare any additional toppings, if desired.

8. When the chicken is cooked, remove on to a chopping board (keep the liquid cooking in the pan) and use two forks to pull the chicken apart into tender strips. Add back into the pan, along with the onions and peppers, and combine everything with the liquid. Continue to cook for 2 minutes until juicy.

9. Make the lime yoghurt by combining the yoghurt alternative and lime juice in a small bowl, stirring well.

10. Warm your tortillas in a stack in the microwave for 30 seconds.

11. Serve all items in bowls on the table for everyone to dig in and create their own fajitas.

STORAGE
Keep everything covered in the fridge for up to 2 days.

Freeze for up to 3 months.

Fish Pie

Tender chunks of iodine-rich fish in a creamy sauce, topped with fluffy mash – for me, this is the ultimate comfort food. It's also a lovely dish to serve guests – when my Canadian mother-in-law first visited, I made this to introduce her to British food. Luckily, she loved it!

EF, GF*, NF, PF, SF*, WF*

Serves: 4 adults and 2 children

Prep: 40 minutes, Cook: 35 minutes

1 leek

1 garlic clove, peeled

1 pack of fish pie mix (340g/12oz) or 4 fillets of skinless, boneless mixed fish (e.g. cod, smoked haddock and salmon)

5g (⅛oz) flat-leaf parsley

1 tbsp oil

50g (1¾oz) butter alternative* or margarine*

50g (1¾oz) plain flour*

500ml (18fl oz) plant-based milk alternative*

1 tsp Dijon mustard (optional)

1 tbsp nutritional yeast

75g (1½oz) frozen peas (or sweetcorn)

juice of ¼ lemon

FOR THE TOPPING

1.25kg (2lb 12oz) floury potatoes (Maris Piper work best)

2 tbsp butter alternative* or margarine*

50ml (2fl oz) plant-based milk alternative*

1. Start by making the topping. Peel and chop the potatoes into big chunks. Add to a large saucepan of boiling water and cook on a medium heat for 18 minutes or until cooked. Drain well, then add the other topping ingredients and mash well until smooth and there are no lumps. Set aside to cool.

2. While the potatoes are cooking, prepare your sauce. Wash the leek, discard the white root and tough green tops, cut lengthways and then slice finely. Dice the garlic. Chop the fish into bite-sized pieces. Finely chop the parsley.

3. In a saucepan, heat the oil on a medium heat, then add the leek and garlic and cook for 3 minutes. Remove on to a plate.

4. Add the butter alternative or margarine into the pan and when melted and bubbling, add the flour and cook, stirring, for 1 minute. Gradually add the milk alternative, whisking constantly, until combined.

5. Add the mustard (if using), nutritional yeast, peas, lemon juice and parsley, stir well and cook for a further minute. Turn off the heat and add the fish chunks, plus the leeks and garlic, folding into the sauce gently.

6. Preheat the oven to 200°C/ Fan 180°C/400°F/Gas Mark 6 while leaving the sauce to cool.

7. Assemble the pie. Pour the sauce into a large ovenproof dish, ensuring the fish is distributed evenly. Take a spoonful of mashed potato at a time and add to the top, starting with the border of the dish, then filling in the middle. Spread out the topping until it's flat and even, ensuring the edges of the dish are sealed.

8. Using the back of a fork, drag it along the topping in a criss-cross pattern to create ridges.

9. Bake in the oven for 30-35 minutes until the edges of the potato are browning.

STORAGE
Keep covered in the fridge for up to 2 days.

Freeze for up to 3 months.

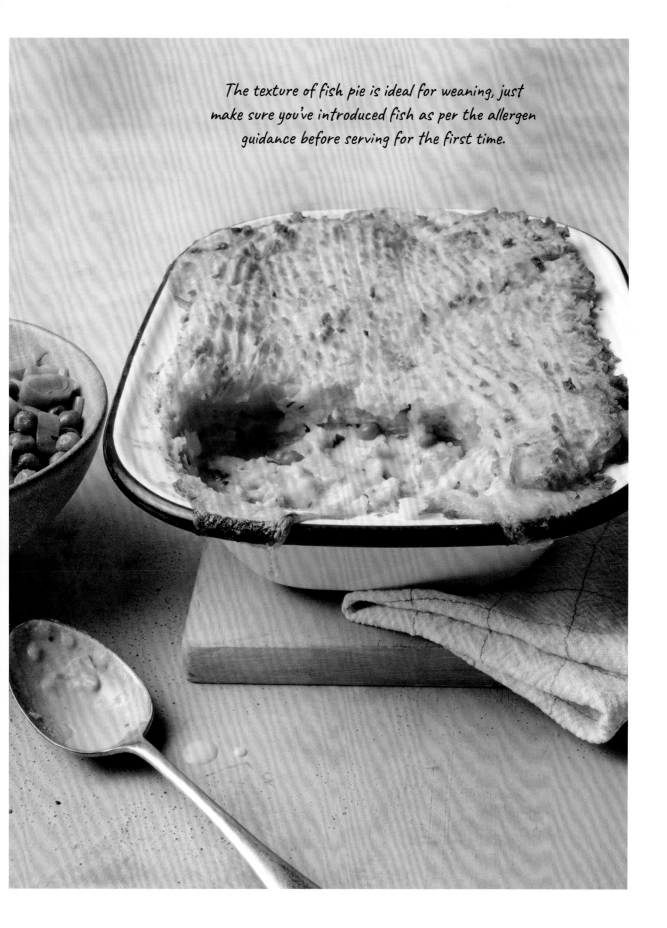

The texture of fish pie is ideal for weaning, just make sure you've introduced fish as per the allergen guidance before serving for the first time.

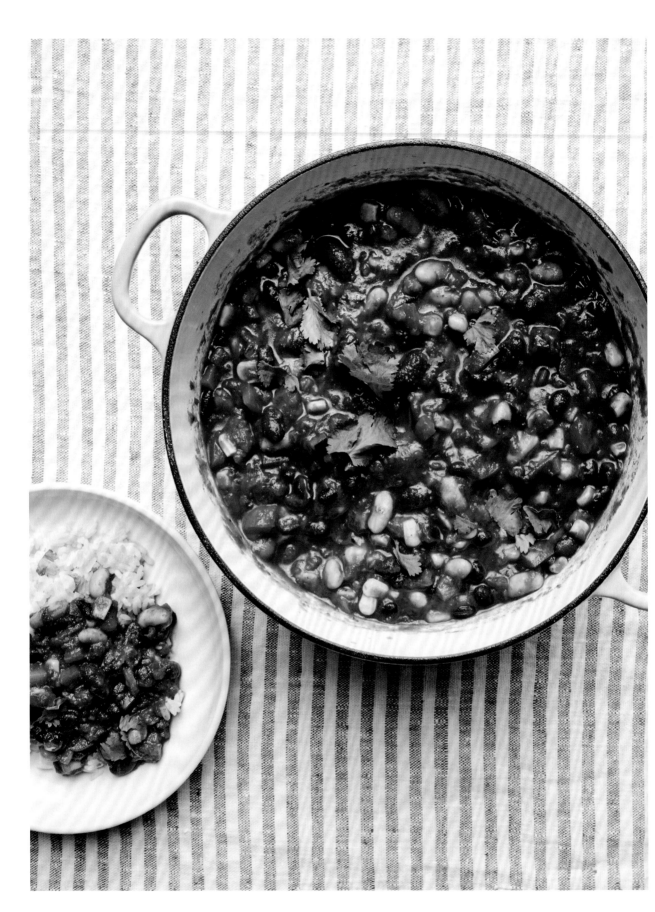

Smoky Three-Bean Chilli

Protein and iron-rich beans with nutritious veggies in a smoky but mild Mexican-inspired sauce. Budget friendly and great for batch cooking – we always have several portions in the freezer stash, as it's requested by the kids at least once a week!

EF, GF*, NF, PF, SF*, V, VG, WF*

Serves: 4 adults and 2 children

Prep: 10 minutes, Cook: 30 minutes

1 onion

2 garlic cloves, peeled

1 red (bell) pepper

½ courgette

spice mix made from: 1 tbsp ground cumin, 2 tbsp smoked paprika, 2 tsp dried oregano, 1 tsp ground coriander

1 tbsp oil

1 tbsp tomato purée

400g (14oz) can chopped tomatoes

300ml (10fl oz) tomato passata

400ml (14fl oz) hot (low-salt) vegetable stock*

400g (14oz) can cannellini or butter beans

400g (14oz) can kidney beans

400g (14oz) can black beans

150g (5½oz) frozen sweetcorn

1 tsp yeast extract spread*, such as Marmite® (optional)

chopped coriander, for garnish

1. Prep your ingredients – dice the onion and garlic, then the red pepper and courgette. Make the spice mix by combining the spices in a bowl and stirring together.

2. In a large saucepan, heat the oil on a low-medium heat, add the onion and garlic and cook, stirring often, for 3 minutes.

3. Add the pepper and courgette, then cook for a further 3 minutes.

4. Add the spice mix and tomato purée, stir well and cook for 1 minute until fragrant.

5. Pour in the chopped tomatoes, passata and hot stock. Bring to the boil, then reduce the heat to low.

6. Drain and rinse all the beans, then add to the pan with the sweetcorn and yeast extract spread (if using). Mix together, then bubble gently for 20-30 minutes until thickened. If too thick, add a splash of water to loosen.

7. Garnish with coriander and serve with fluffy rice. I tend to separate the adult portions into a separate pan once cooked, then add additional spices and some chilli powder for an extra kick.

STORAGE
Keep covered in the fridge for up to 3 days.

Freeze for up to 6 months.

Yeast extract spread is typically salty, but you can buy low-salt and gluten-free versions now. When used sparingly in recipes like this it can add a lovely depth of flavour.
Squash the beans with the back of a fork for babies and younger children before serving.

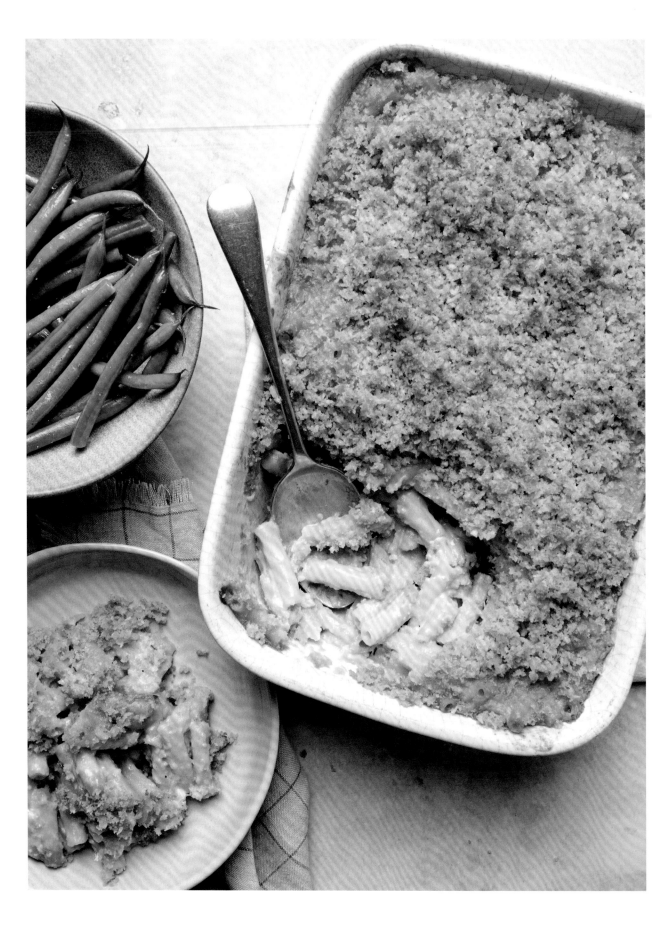

Baked Mac 'n' Cheeze

Another highly requested recipe, and no wonder. It's such a family classic, but one you'd be forgiven for assuming you couldn't make dairy free. Not true! This is so creamy and satisfying, with a gorgeously crispy topping. The leftovers don't last long with me around!

EF, GF*, NF, PF, SF*, V, VG, WF*

Serves: 4 adults and 2 children

Prep: 25 minutes, Cook: 30 minutes

250g (9oz) macaroni*

1 tbsp butter alternative* or margarine*

FOR THE SAUCE

80g (2¾oz) Cheddar alternative*

90g (3¼oz) butter alternative* or margarine*

75g (2½oz) plain flour*

700ml (1¼ pints) plant-based milk alternative*

4 tbsp nutritional yeast

½ tsp Dijon mustard (optional)

freshly ground black pepper

FOR THE TOPPING

2 tbsp butter alternative* or margarine*

75g (2½oz) panko breadcrumbs* (or gluten-free breadcrumbs)

40g (1½oz) Cheddar alternative*

1. Preheat the oven to 200°C/Fan 180°C/400°F/Gas Mark 6.

2. In a large saucepan of boiling water, cook the macaroni for 2 minutes less than the packet instructions, then drain and add the butter alternative or margarine. Stir well and set aside. This helps to stop the pasta becoming stodgy when baked.

3. Meanwhile, make your sauce. Firstly, grate the Cheddar alternative with a fine grater.

4. In a saucepan, melt the butter alternative or margarine on a medium heat until bubbling. Add the flour and cook, stirring, for 1 minute.

5. Add the milk alternative gradually, whisking constantly until it is all absorbed.

6. Add the nutritional yeast, mustard (if using), grated Cheddar alternative and a crack of black pepper, then stir until combined.

7. Combine with the macaroni, stir together, then pour into a large ovenproof dish.

8. To make the topping, melt the butter alternative or margarine, then add to a bowl with the breadcrumbs and grated Cheddar alternative. Mix well with a spoon until combined, then sprinkle evenly over the macaroni.

9. Bake in the oven for 30 minutes until golden.

10. Serve with green vegetables or salad.

STORAGE

Keep covered in the fridge for up to 3 days.

Freeze for up to 6 months.

I find a 'smoky' version of a Cheddar alternative works really well in this recipe. If you're a fan of spice, drizzle some hot sauce on top of adult portions – delicious!

'No Butter' Chicken

A perfect weekend fakeaway, this version of a popular classic curry is delicious. The sauce is mild enough for all ages, but I've also included some optional extras if you want to ramp up the flavour.

EF, GF*, NF*, PF, SF*, WF*

Serves: 2 adults and 2 children

Prep: 10 minutes, Cook: 20 minutes

FOR THE CHICKEN AND MARINADE

3 chicken breasts or 500g (1lb 2oz) diced chicken

1 tsp ginger paste

1 tsp garlic paste

2 tsp ground cumin

1 tbsp garam masala

½ tsp ground turmeric

120g (4¼oz) plain Greek-style yoghurt alternative*

FOR COOKING

1 tbsp butter alternative* or margarine*

1 tbsp oil

FOR THE SAUCE

150ml (5fl oz) tomato passata

200ml (7fl oz) cream alternative*

1 tbsp plain Greek-style yoghurt alternative*

OPTIONAL EXTRAS

ground almonds*

desiccated coconut

chopped coriander

sliced red chillies

1. Chop the chicken into bite-sized pieces, then add to a bowl with the marinade ingredients and mix well until all the chicken is coated. Set aside.

2. Heat the oil and butter alternative or margarine in a large, non-stick saucepan on a high heat. When bubbling, add the chicken and cook, stirring often, for 5–6 minutes until sealed on all sides.

3. Add the passata, bring to the boil, then reduce the heat to low.

4. Stir in the cream and yoghurt alternatives, then simmer for 10 minutes until the sauce is thickened and the chicken is cooked through.

5. Serve with basmati rice, topping with a sprinkle of the optional extras if desired.

STORAGE
Keep covered in the fridge for up to 3 days.

Freeze for up to 6 months.

Add bell peppers, peas or chopped green beans into the curry for added nutrition or serve with veg on the side.
If you have time, refrigerate the marinated chicken for a few hours (or overnight) to intensify the flavour.

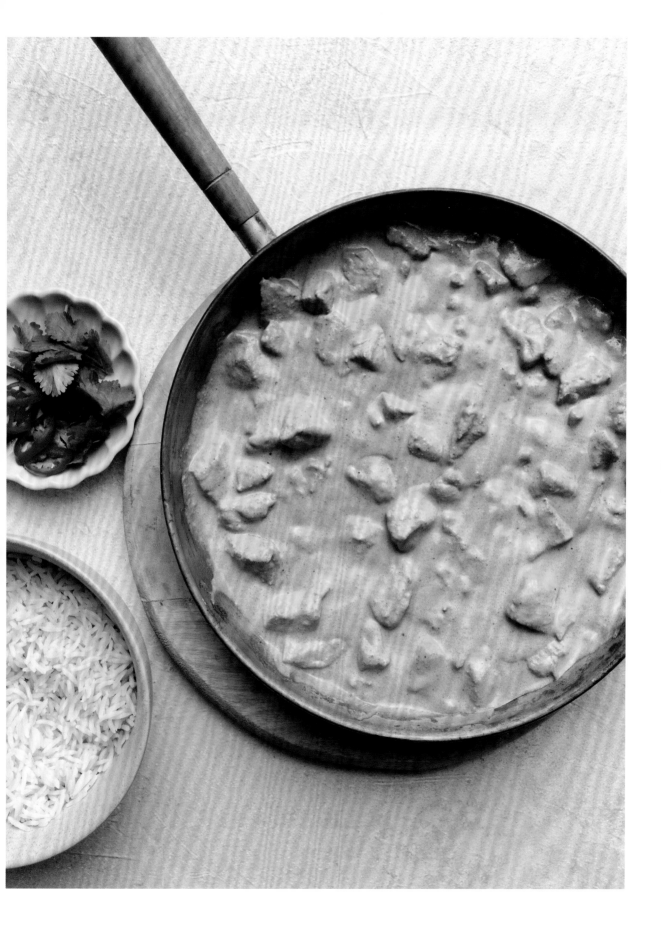

Fish Goujons *with a* Couscous Crust

This is my twist on fish fingers - couscous makes for such a lovely, crispy crust. Firm white fish (cod, basa, hake or haddock) works well and is high in iodine, or you could also use salmon. Swap the couscous for quinoa for a gluten-free alternative.

GF*, NF, PF, SF, WF*

Serves: 2 adults and 2 children

Prep: 15 minutes, Cook: 12 minutes

75g (2½oz) couscous* (or quinoa)

½ tsp dried parsley

juice of ½ lemon

200g (7oz) skinless white fish fillets

3 tbsp plain flour*

1 egg

1. Preheat the oven to 200°C/ Fan 180°C/400°F/Gas Mark 6 and line a large oven tray with baking paper.

2. To a large bowl, add the couscous, parsley and lemon juice. Mix well, then add 75ml (2½fl oz) boiling water, stir and cover with a plate for 5 minutes until the water is absorbed. Fluff with a fork.

3. Meanwhile, cut your fish into large strips.

4. Add the flour to a bowl, and in a separate bowl beat the egg.

5. Dip each piece of fish into the flour on both sides, then dunk into the beaten egg. Finally, lower into the couscous, using your fingers to press the couscous into the fish until fully coated on all sides. Place on to the prepared oven tray.

6. Repeat for all the fish pieces, then bake for 10-12 minutes until crispy and the fish is cooked through.

7. Serve with your favourite style of potatoes and veg.

STORAGE
Keep covered in the fridge for up to 1 day.

Not suitable for freezing.

Add the zest of the lemon to the couscous for an extra zing.

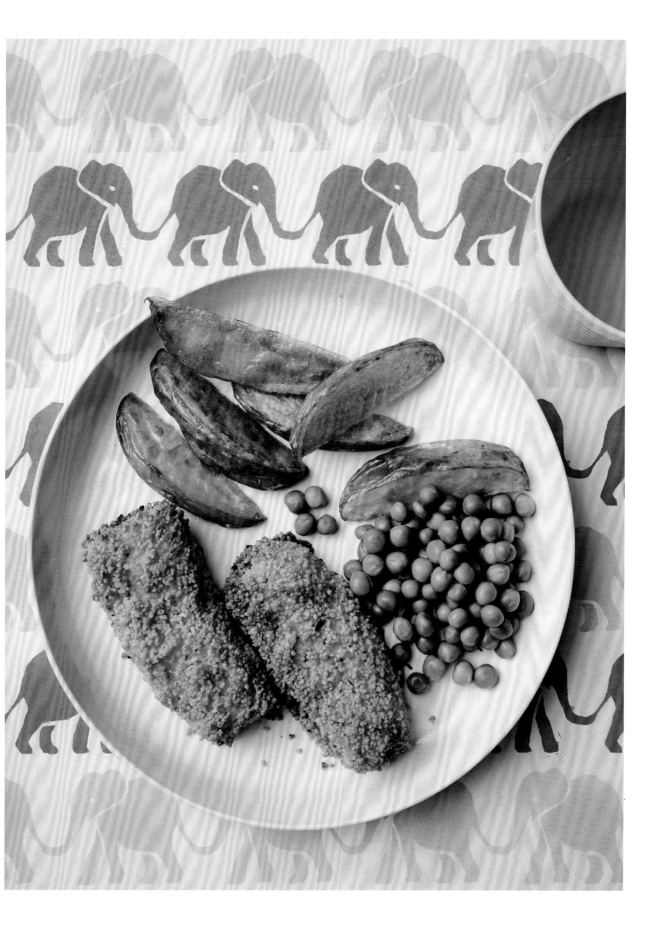

One-Pot

If you've followed my Instagram for a while, you'll know that I love a one-pot recipe. Mainly because I hate washing up, but also because I find something so satisfying about serving your family from one dish. Why not place it in the middle of the table and let the adults and bigger kids help themselves?

Coconut Lentil Dhal

Protein-rich lentils meet creamy coconut and warming spices in this easy plant-based dish. Ideal for all ages from weaning onwards, I usually separate the adults' portions and add some extra curry powder and chilli plus fresh coriander leaves for a further flavour boost.

EF, GF*, NF, PF, SF*, V, VG, WF*

Serves: 2 adults and 2 children

Prep: 10 minutes, Cook: 20 minutes

1 onion

2 garlic cloves, peeled (or 1 tbsp garlic paste)

2.5cm (1in) piece of fresh ginger (or 1 tbsp ginger paste)

200g (7oz) split red lentils

1 tbsp oil

1 tsp tomato purée

1 tbsp mild curry powder

1 tsp ground coriander

½ tsp ground turmeric

400ml (14oz) hot (low-salt) vegetable stock*

400g (14oz) can coconut milk

1. Prep your ingredients - dice the onion and garlic, peel and dice or grate the ginger.

2. Rinse the lentils in a sieve under cold water for 2 minutes, swirling and rubbing between your fingers.

3. Heat the oil in a large saucepan on a low-medium heat, then add the onion, garlic and ginger and cook, stirring often, for 3 minutes.

4. Add the tomato purée, curry powder, ground coriander and turmeric, stir well and cook for a further minute until fragrant.

5. Add the lentils, hot stock and coconut milk, bring to the boil, then reduce the heat to low and cook, uncovered, for 15 minutes, stirring regularly. Serve.

STORAGE
Keep covered in the fridge for up to 3 days.

Freeze for up to 6 months.

Double the quantities and freeze leftovers for an easy meal on busy days.

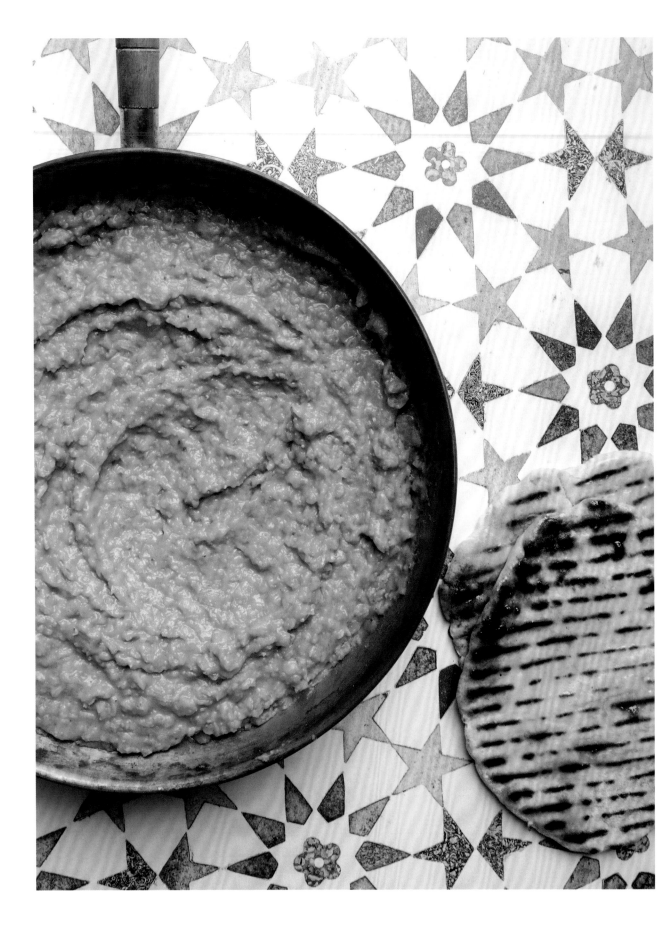

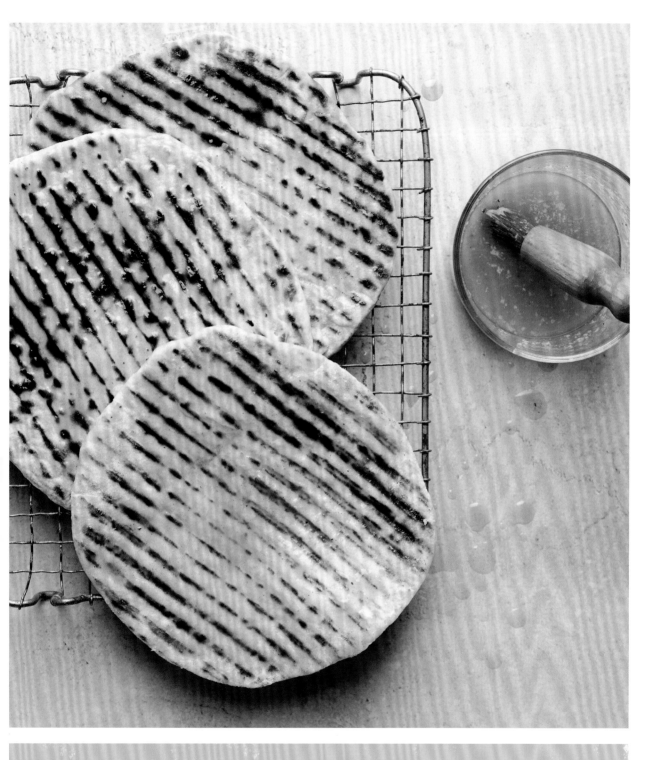

Why not make some homemade naan to dunk? Follow my Two-Ingredient Dough recipe on page 155, shape into oval/flatbread shapes and cook in a lightly oiled frying pan, or griddle pan for 2 minutes on each side. You could even add some garlic butter too (just add garlic paste to some melted butter alternative)!

Sausage Traybake

Deliciously simple, this has been one of my favourite recipes for years. A quick bit of prep and then the oven does all the hard work!

EF, GF*, NF, PF, SF*, WF*

Serves: 2 adults and 2 children

Prep: 10-15 minutes, Cook: 55 minutes

2 red onions

1 red (bell) pepper

200g (7oz) cherry or plum tomatoes (approx. 16)

2 garlic cloves, peeled

500g (1lb 2oz) baby new potatoes

8 good-quality sausages*

1½ tbsp oil

150ml (5fl oz) hot (low-salt) beef, chicken or vegetable stock*

chopped flat-leaf parsley, to serve

1. Preheat the oven to 200°C/Fan 180°C/400°F/Gas Mark 6.

2. Prep your veg - slice the red onion and red pepper into thin wedges. Cut the cherry tomatoes in half. Finely dice the garlic. Wash and dry the potatoes and cut into 2.5cm (1in) pieces.

3. Place the sausages, onions, pepper, garlic, tomatoes, potatoes and oil into a large roasting dish. Toss together so everything is coated with the oil. Distribute the ingredients in one layer, with the sausages evenly spread around the dish.

4. Bake in the oven for 35 minutes.

5. Remove the sausages on to a plate and stir the veg. Pour the hot stock into the dish, then stir again, scraping any sticky bits off the bottom until everything is coated with the stock. Replace the sausages but turn on to the other side.

6. Put the dish back into the oven for a further 15-20 minutes until the sausages are brown and the potatoes are golden.

STORAGE

Keep covered in the fridge for up to 2 days.

Not suitable for freezing.

Any sausages can be used – vegetarian, chicken or low salt, but you may need to adjust the cooking time accordingly.

Make sure your roasting dish is large enough so that everything is spread on one layer. If you have a smaller dish, the potatoes may not cook through properly, so consider splitting ingredients over two dishes.

Avoid cutting sausages into coin shapes for children as this is a choking hazard; instead cut lengthways first, then into small pieces.

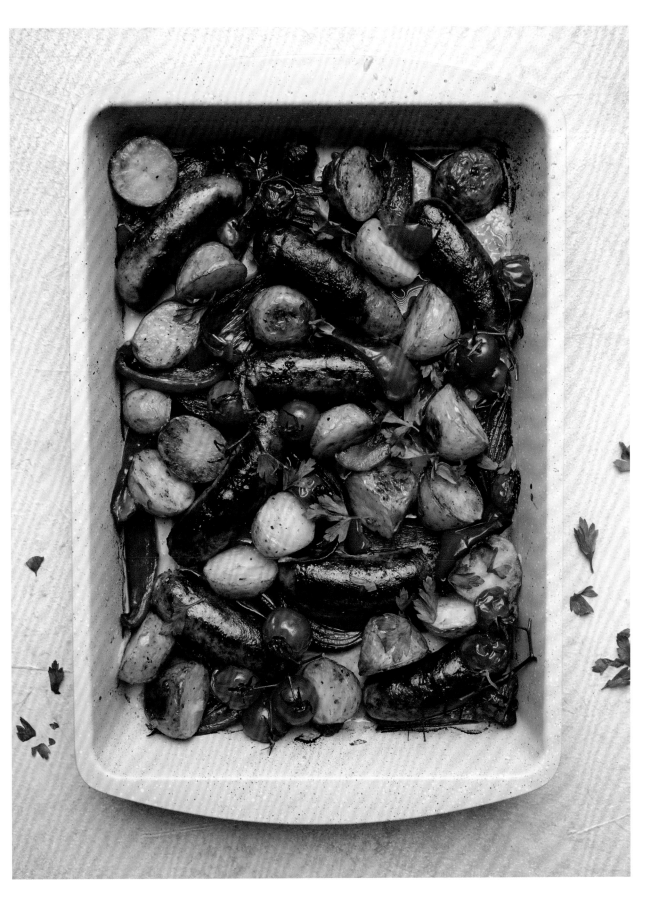

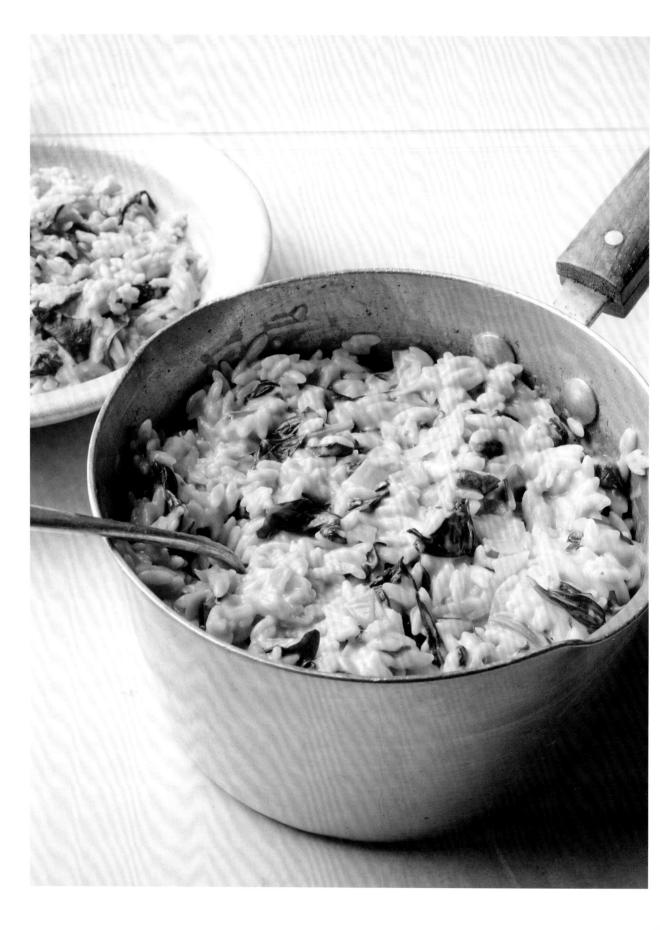

Cheezy Leek & Spinach Orzo

Creamy and comforting, with the added goodness of green veg. Orzo is a great pasta for weaning and young kids, as the small shape makes it easy to scoop. This dish will be a hit with everyone at the table though.

EF, NF, PF, SF*, V, VG

Serves: 2 adults and 2 children

Prep: 8 minutes, Cook: 22 minutes

1 leek

1 garlic clove, peeled

100g (3½oz) baby spinach leaves

100g (3½oz) Cheddar alternative*

1 tbsp oil

300g (10½oz) orzo pasta

700ml (1¼ pints) hot (low-salt) vegetable stock*

150ml (5fl oz) plant-based milk alternative*

zest and juice of 1 lemon

1. Prep your ingredients - wash and dice the leek, discarding the roots and tough green tops. Finely dice or grate the garlic. Chop the spinach roughly. Finely grate the Cheddar alternative.

2. In a large, lidded saucepan, heat the oil on a medium heat. Add the leek and cook for 3-4 minutes, stirring often, until softened. Then add the garlic for a further minute.

3. Add the orzo and cook, stirring, for 1 minute until coated in the oil.

4. Add the hot stock and milk alternative, stir and bring to the boil.

5. Cover the pan with its lid, reduce the heat to low and simmer for 12 minutes, stirring every couple of minutes.

6. Add the spinach to the pan along with the lemon zest and juice, stir well, then cover the pan for another 2 minutes until the orzo is cooked.

7. Remove from the heat and stir through the grated Cheddar alternative until combined, then serve.

STORAGE
Keep covered in the fridge for up to 2 days.

Freeze for up to 3 months.

Spinach can be swapped for peas or other veg if preferred.

Spanish Prawn & Chorizo Rice

I've stopped short of calling this a paella, but it's got similar flavour vibes. Smoky chorizo, juicy prawns and mildly spiced rice make for a wonderfully tasty meal. Double check the chorizo is dairy free, as not all is!

EF, GF*, NF, PF, SF*, WF*

Serves: 2 adults and 2 children (with leftovers)

Prep: 10 minutes, Cook: 25 minutes

50g (1¾oz) chorizo ring*

1 onion

2 (bell) peppers (I use red and yellow)

2 garlic cloves, peeled

spice mix made from: 1 tbsp smoked paprika, 1 tbsp ground coriander, 1 tsp garlic powder, 2 tsp ground cumin, 1 tsp dried parsley

300g (10½oz) basmati rice

1 tbsp oil

165g (5¾oz) raw king prawns

600ml (20fl oz) hot (low-salt) chicken stock*

400g (14oz) can chopped tomatoes

150g (5½oz) frozen peas (or sweetcorn)

juice of ½ lemon

1. Prep your ingredients - chop the chorizo into small pieces and set aside. Dice the onion, peppers and garlic. Put the spice mix ingredients into a bowl and stir together.

2. Rinse the rice in a sieve under cold water for 2 minutes, swirling with your hands.

3. Heat the oil in a large, lidded non-stick pan on a medium heat, add the chorizo and cook for 3 minutes until starting to crisp, then add the prawns, stirring until pink all over.

4. Remove the chorizo and prawns on to a plate, reserving the oil in the pan.

5. Add the onion, peppers and garlic to the pan and cook for 4 minutes, stirring often.

6. Add the spice mix, stir well and cook for a further minute, then add the rinsed rice, hot stock and chopped tomatoes.

7. Stir, bring to the boil, then cover the pan with its lid, reduce the heat to low and simmer for 12-14 minutes, stirring every few minutes (making sure nothing is stuck to the bottom of the pan) until the rice is nearly cooked.

8. Add the peas, stir well, cover with the lid and cook for a further 2 minutes.

9. Add the chorizo and prawns back into the pan, along with the lemon juice, then mix well until all heated through. Serve.

STORAGE
Keep covered in the fridge for up to 2 days. Don't reheat rice more than once.

Not suitable for freezing.

Chorizo is salty, so if serving to infants leave out the chorizo pieces from their plate – they can still get some of the flavour from the oil the rice is cooked in. Prawns are an allergen (crustacean) so follow guidance when introducing for the first time (see page 50) and also ensure they are completely cooked through.

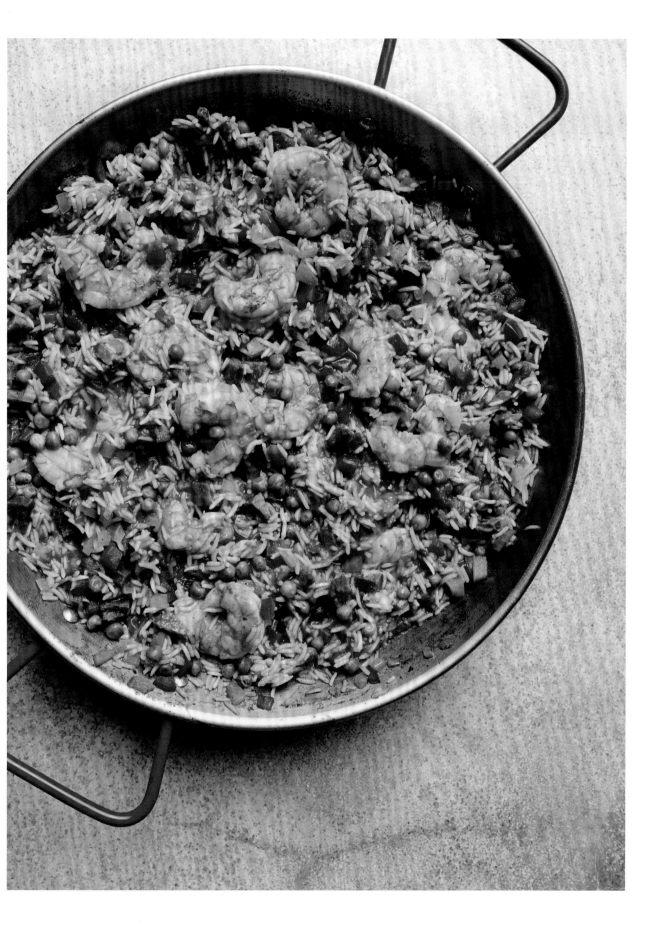

'Bung it all in' Chicken Casserole

This earns its name because you can basically bung in whatever veg you have in the fridge, and bonus... there's no pre-cooking! The result is beautifully tender chicken. This dish is delicious on its own, or if you wanted to stretch it further you could serve it with mashed potato or rice.

EF, GF*, NF, PF, SF*, WF*

Serves: 4 adults and 2 children

Prep: 25 minutes, Cook: 1 hour

2 onions

2 carrots

2 celery sticks

1 butternut squash (or 2 small, sweet potatoes), peeled

2 garlic cloves, peeled

600g (1lb 5oz) boneless, skinless chicken thighs

2 (low-salt) chicken stock cubes*

1 tbsp Dijon mustard (optional)

1 tbsp dried mixed herbs

400g (14oz) can butter beans

2 tbsp cornflour

chopped flat-leaf parsley, to serve

1. Preheat the oven to 190°C/ Fan 170°C/375°F/Gas Mark 5.

2. Roughly chop the onions, carrots, celery and butternut squash. Finely dice the garlic.

3. Put all the ingredients, except the butter beans and cornflour, into a large, lidded casserole pot, along with 500ml (18fl oz) boiling water. Stir well, then cover with the lid. Cook in the oven for 45 minutes.

4. Remove a few spoonfuls of the cooking liquid into a small bowl and stir in the cornflour until it makes a thick paste, then stir that into the casserole.

5. Drain and rinse the beans and add in, stir well and cover with the lid again, cooking for a further 15 minutes.

6. Serve in bowls, topped with the flat-leaf parsley.

STORAGE

Keep covered in the fridge for up to 3 days.

Freeze for up to 3 months.

Cooking chicken in this way is ideal for weaning; offer in strips for baby to hold.
This can also be cooked in a slow cooker, for 3–4 hours on high or 7 hours on low, then a further 30 minutes with the cornflour and beans.

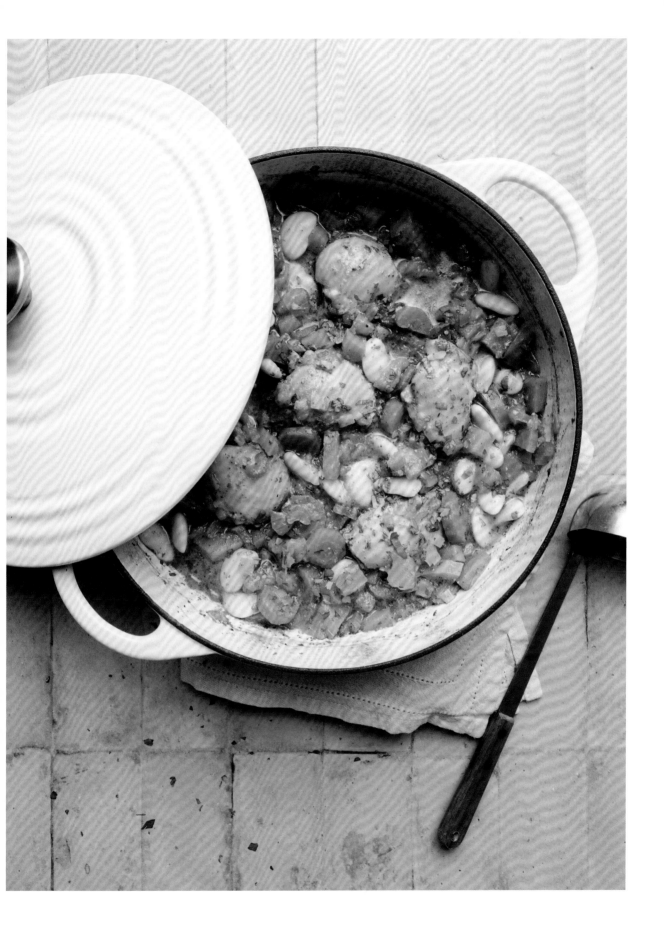

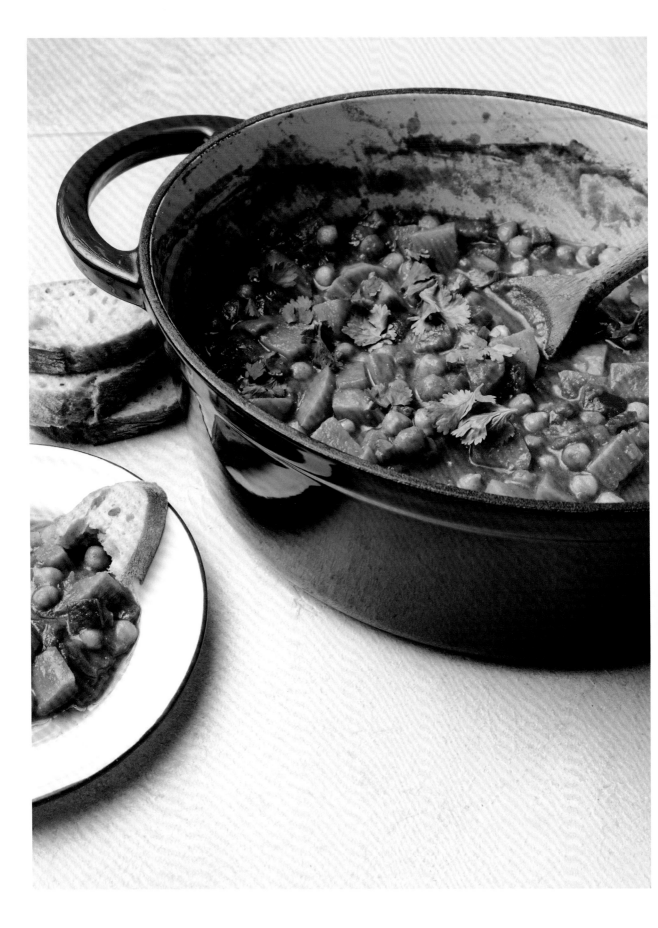

Sweet Potato & Chickpea Stew

A warming plant-based stew with a hearty and nutritious tomato and peanut butter sauce. This is a great one for batch cooking and having in the freezer stash. Serve in a bowl with crusty bread to dip.

EF, GF*, NF, SF*, V, VG, WF*

Serves: 2 adults and 2 children

Prep: 10 minutes, Cook: 40 minutes

1 onion

2 garlic cloves, peeled

1 red (bell) pepper

250g (9oz) sweet potatoes

1 tbsp oil

1 tsp ground smoked paprika

1 tbsp ground cumin

¼ tsp ground cinnamon

1 tbsp tomato purée

500ml (18fl oz) hot (low-salt) vegetable stock*

50g (1¾oz) smooth peanut butter

400g (14oz) can chopped tomatoes

400g (14oz) can chickpeas

coriander leaves, to serve (optional)

1. Prep your ingredients - dice the onion, garlic and pepper. Peel the sweet potatoes and chop into 1cm (½in) cubes.

2. In a large saucepan, heat the oil on a medium heat, then add the onion and cook for 3 minutes. Add the garlic and cook for a further minute.

3. Add the pepper and sweet potato, stir and cook for 3 minutes, then add the smoked paprika, cumin, cinnamon and tomato purée and cook for a further 2 minutes.

4. Meanwhile, mix the hot stock with the peanut butter in a jug, then add to the pan along with the chopped tomatoes.

5. Bring to the boil, then reduce the heat to low and simmer for 20-25 minutes, stirring every few minutes.

6. Drain and rinse the chickpeas and add to the pan. Cook for a further 5-10 minutes.

7. Serve, garnished with coriander.

STORAGE
Keep covered in the fridge for up to 3 days.

Freeze for up to 6 months.

Omit the chickpeas if you have a legume allergy, and replace with extra veg like aubergine, spinach or kale.
For babies and younger children, whole chickpeas can be a choking hazard, so mash gently with the back of a fork to serve.

Speedy Suppers

All the recipes in this book are simple, but if you're short on time and still want something delicious for dinner, that's where speedy suppers come in. All of these meals are ready in 30 minutes or less. You'll also find some of my favourite 'cheat' hacks in there too, which are helpful to have in your back pocket for lazy days.

Thai Coconut Chicken Noodles

Ever since I went travelling to Southeast Asia, Thai has been my favourite cuisine. It's not always child-friendly, but this easy sauce has delicious, fragrant flavours without the fiery chilli kick for kids. I do love adding some sriracha to the adult portions when serving though!

EF, GF*, NF, PF, SF*, WF*

Serves: 2 adults and 2 children

Prep: 10-15 minutes, Cook: 15 minutes

1 red (bell) pepper

125g (4½oz) green beans

100g (3½oz) broccoli florets

200g (7oz) rice noodles (pad Thai-style ones work best)

1 tbsp oil

500g (1lb 2oz) chicken breast strips (or diced)

coriander leaves (optional)

lime for garnish (optional)

FOR THE SAUCE

300ml (10fl oz) canned coconut milk (shake well before use)

1 tsp ginger paste

2 tsp garlic paste

1 tsp lemongrass paste

2 tbsp low-salt soy sauce* or soya-free coconut aminos*

juice of 1 lime

1 tsp fish sauce (optional)

1½ tsp maple syrup (not required if using coconut aminos)

¼ tsp chilli flakes (optional)

1. First, prepare your sauce. Add all the ingredients to a bowl and stir for a minute to combine. Taste and adjust the flavours as you wish by adding more of the different ingredients. The aim is to get a balance of creamy, sour, sweet and salty.

2. Top and tail the green beans, then cut into 2.5cm (1in) pieces. Slice the pepper into thin strips and chop the broccoli florets into bite-sized pieces.

3. Cook the rice noodles as per the packet instructions and drain. Meanwhile, cook your stir fry.

4. In a large wok or saucepan, heat the oil on a high heat, then add the chicken. Cook for 3-4 minutes, stirring regularly, until coloured on all sides.

5. Add the pepper, green beans and broccoli and continue to cook, stirring often, for another 5 minutes until the chicken and veg are cooked.

6. Pour in the sauce and cook for 1 minute, then add the drained noodles, toss together to combine.

7. Serve, garnishing with torn coriander leaves and slices of lime if you wish.

STORAGE
Keep covered in the fridge for up to 1 day.

Not suitable for freezing.

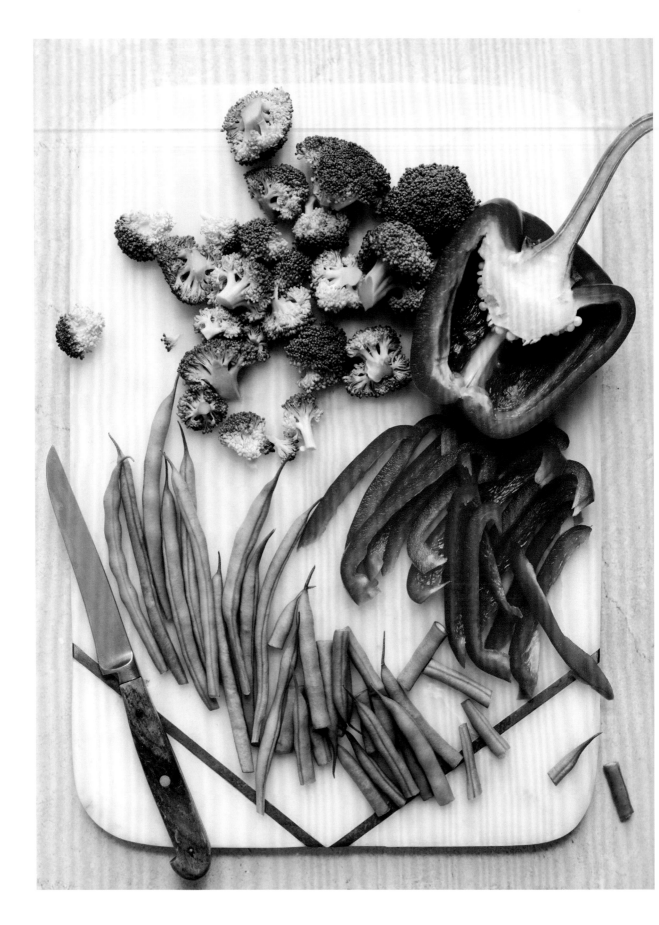

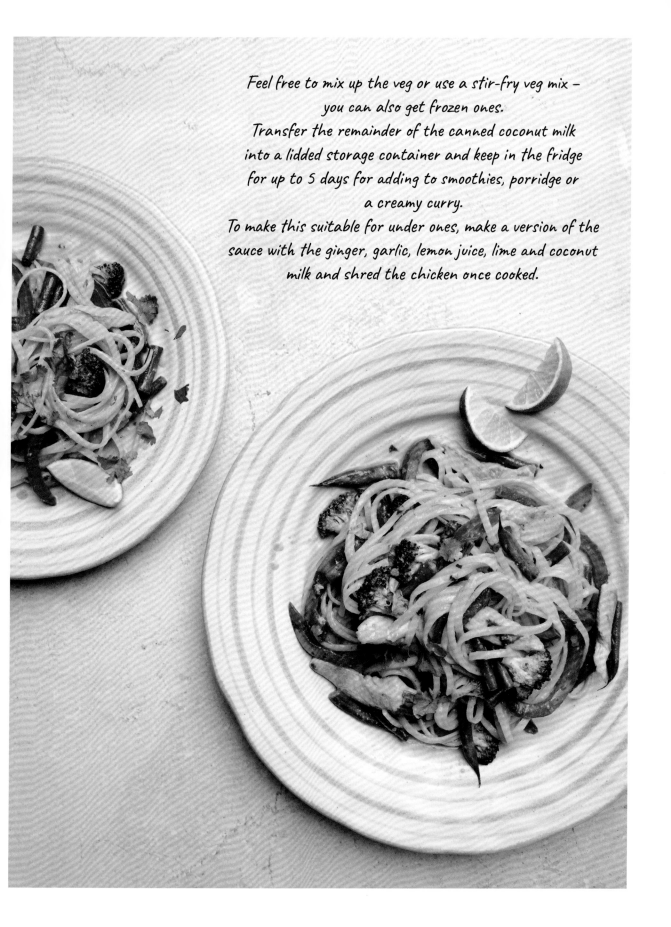

Feel free to mix up the veg or use a stir-fry veg mix —
you can also get frozen ones.
Transfer the remainder of the canned coconut milk
into a lidded storage container and keep in the fridge
for up to 5 days for adding to smoothies, porridge or
a creamy curry.
To make this suitable for under ones, make a version of the
sauce with the ginger, garlic, lemon juice, lime and coconut
milk and shred the chicken once cooked.

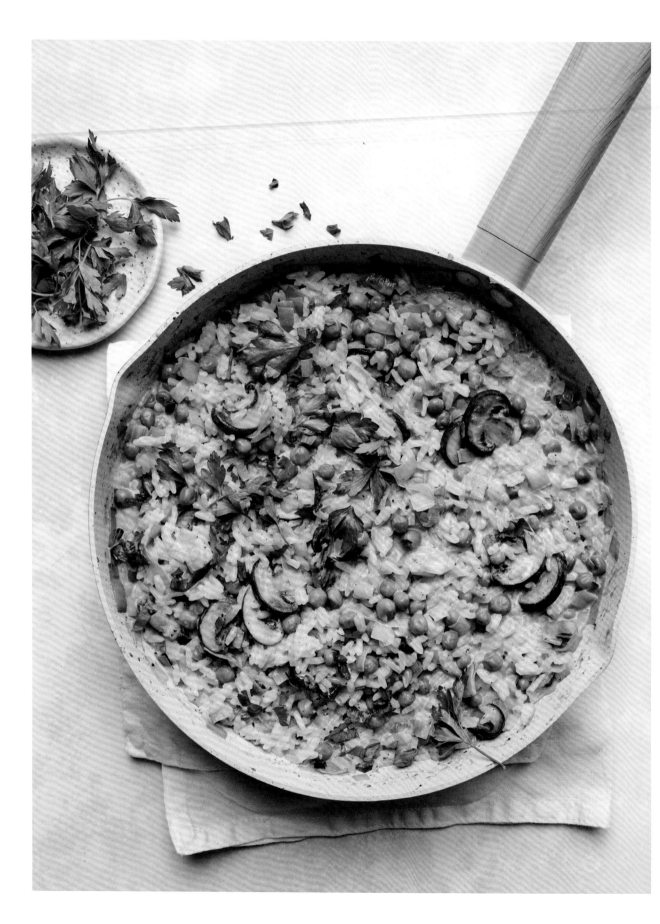

Cheat Spring Green Risotto

My cheat risottos are a real hit with my followers, so here's a new version using some of my favourite spring veggies. Granted, it may not be for risotto purists, but the hack of using microwave rice means it's on the table in 20 minutes and is so creamy and delicious, without the usual arm ache of stirring a proper risotto!

EF, GF*, NF, PF, SF*, V, VG, WF*

Serves: 2 adults and 2 children

Prep: 10 minutes, Cook: 10 minutes

1 leek

1 handful of mushrooms

150g (5½oz) frozen peas

1 tbsp oil

2 tsp garlic paste

120ml (4fl oz) hot (low-salt) vegetable stock*

4 tbsp soft cheese alternative*

2 x 250g (9oz) pouches of microwavable long-grain rice

juice of ½ lemon

100ml (3½fl oz) cream alternative*, plus extra to loosen if needed

4 tbsp nutritional yeast

1 tsp dried mixed herbs

flat-leaf parsley, to serve (optional)

1. Prep your ingredients – wash and dice the leek, discarding the white root and tough green tops. Wash and slice the mushrooms. Add the peas to a bowl of boiling water to start defrosting.

2. In a large saucepan, heat the oil on a medium heat, then add the garlic paste, leek and mushrooms. Cook, stirring often, for 3 minutes until softened.

3. Drain and add the peas, along with the hot stock and soft cheese alternative, then stir until melted and combined.

4. Before opening the rice pouches, break up the grains with your fingers, then open the packs and add to the pan with the lemon juice, cream alternative, nutritional yeast and herbs.

5. Stir well and cook for 2 minutes, ensuring the peas are cooked through. Add a splash more cream alternative to loosen if needed.

6. Serve, topped with chopped flat-leaf parsley if you wish.

STORAGE
Keep covered in the fridge for up to 1 day. Refrigerate as soon as cooled and reheat until piping hot. Never reheat rice more than once.

Not suitable for freezing.

*Any vegetables can be used, so raid the fridge or freezer!
If you're a meat eater, you can add cooked, chopped chicken for added protein,
or if you're vegetarian, then chickpeas would also work well.*

Creamy Mustard Pork
with Cheat Mash

My partner Mike's favourite ever dish is *porc à la moutarde* (pork with mustard), so I had to create a dairy-free version. So delicious and comforting, perfect for colder nights. Cheat mash uses baking potatoes but feel free to make traditional mash, or serve with crispy oven-baked or air-fryer potatoes.

EF, GF*, NF, PF, SF*, WF*

Serves: 2 adults and 2 children

Prep: 10 minutes, Cook: 20 minutes

1 leek

1 garlic clove, peeled

4 pork loin steaks or 500g (1lb 2oz) diced pork topside

1 tbsp oil

150ml (5fl oz) hot (low-salt) chicken stock*

1 tbsp Dijon mustard

2 tsp wholegrain mustard

1 tsp dried parsley

150ml (5fl oz) cream alternative*

1 tsp cornflour

FOR THE CHEAT MASH

700g (1lb 9oz) baking potatoes

1 tbsp butter alternative* or margarine*

2 tbsp plant-based milk alternative*

1. First, cook your potatoes for the cheat mash. Wash, then dry the potatoes and prick each one several times all over with a fork. Place on a large microwavable plate and microwave for 18 minutes, turning over once halfway, then leave to cool.

2. Meanwhile, cook the sauce. Wash and dice the leeks, discarding the white root and tough green tops. Finely dice the garlic. Chop the pork into 2.5cm (1in) pieces.

3. In a large saucepan, heat the oil on high, add the pork and fry for 2 minutes on each side. Remove on to a plate, reserving the fat in the pan.

4. Turn the heat down to low–medium, add the leek and garlic and cook for 2–3 minutes.

5. Add the hot stock, bring to the boil, then reduce the heat to low and simmer for 5 minutes.

6. Add the two types of mustard, stir for 1 minute, then add the cream alternative and parsley and stir.

7. Pour the cornflour into a small bowl, then add several spoonfuls of the mustard sauce and stir well to combine. Add the mixture to the pan and stir well.

8. Add the pork back into the pan, along with any resting juices, and simmer for 5 minutes until cooked.

9. Meanwhile, finish the potatoes and cook any vegetables for the side. Carefully cut the potatoes (they'll be very hot!) and scoop out the flesh into a large bowl, add the butter alternative or margarine and milk alternative and mash together.

10. Serve the sauce on top of the potatoes, with a side of green veg.

STORAGE
Keep covered in the fridge for up to 2 days.

Freeze the pork for up to 3 months.

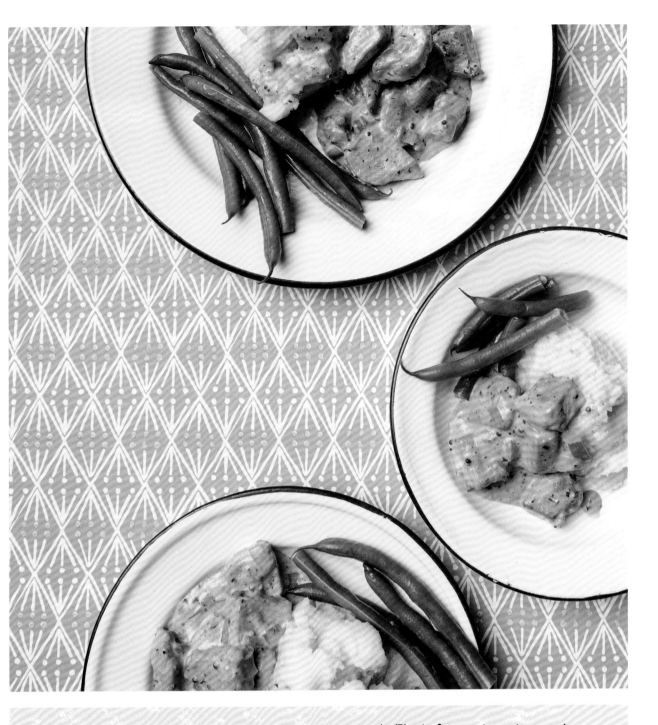

The key is not to overcook or dry out your pork. Flash-frying it, resting and then letting it simmer in the sauce makes it lovely and tender – just ensure it is cooked through before serving.

For weaning, offer strips of the pork to hold, and remember mustard is an allergen, so make sure you follow guidance on introducing it for the first time before serving this dish.

Turkish-Style Lamb & Aubergine Stew *with* Couscous

Warming Middle Eastern spices combine so well with tender lamb mince and aubergine in this tasty dish. When I first made it, Violet said 'This is DEFINITELY going in the book!' So there you go... the ultimate accolade!

EF, NF, PF, SF*

Serves: 2 adults and 2 children

Prep: 10 minutes, Cook: 20 minutes

1 red onion (use frozen to speed up the prep time)

1 garlic clove, peeled (or 1 tsp garlic paste)

1 ripe tomato

1 aubergine

spice mix made from: 2 tsp ground cumin, 1 tsp paprika, 1 tsp ground coriander, ¼ tsp ground cinnamon

1 tbsp oil

250g (9oz) minced lamb

300ml (10fl oz) hot (low-salt) chicken or beef stock*

2 tbsp tomato purée

FOR THE COUSCOUS

200g (7oz) couscous

300ml (10fl oz) hot (low-salt) chicken or vegetable stock*

juice of ½ lemon

1 tbsp olive oil

FOR THE CUCUMBER 'YOGHURT'

5cm (2in) piece of cucumber

5 tbsp plain Greek-style yoghurt alternative*

juice of ¼ lemon

1. Prep the ingredients for the stew - dice the red onion, garlic and tomato. Chop the aubergine into bite-sized pieces. Make the spice mix by combining the ingredients in a bowl and stirring together.

2. In a large saucepan, heat the oil on a medium heat, then add the onion and garlic and cook, stirring, for 3 minutes.

3. Add the aubergine and cook for a further 4-5 minutes, stirring often.

4. Add the tomato and spices, cooking for 1 minute until fragrant.

5. Add the lamb and cook for a few minutes until brown, breaking up any larger pieces with a wooden spoon.

6. Pour in the hot stock and tomato purée, stir and bring to the boil, then reduce the heat to low and simmer for 5-10 minutes while you prepare the couscous and cucumber 'yoghurt'.

7. Add the couscous to a heatproof bowl, pour in the hot stock and lemon juice, stir and cover with a plate for 5 minutes. Then add the olive oil and fluff with a fork.

8. Coarsely grate the cucumber, then squeeze out the excess water with a clean tea towel. Add the cucumber to a small bowl with the yoghurt alternative and lemon juice, then mix well.

9. Serve the stew on top of the couscous, with the cucumber 'yoghurt' on the side.

STORAGE
Keep covered in the fridge for up to 2 days.

Stew can be frozen for up to 3 months. Cucumber 'yoghurt' is not suitable for freezing.

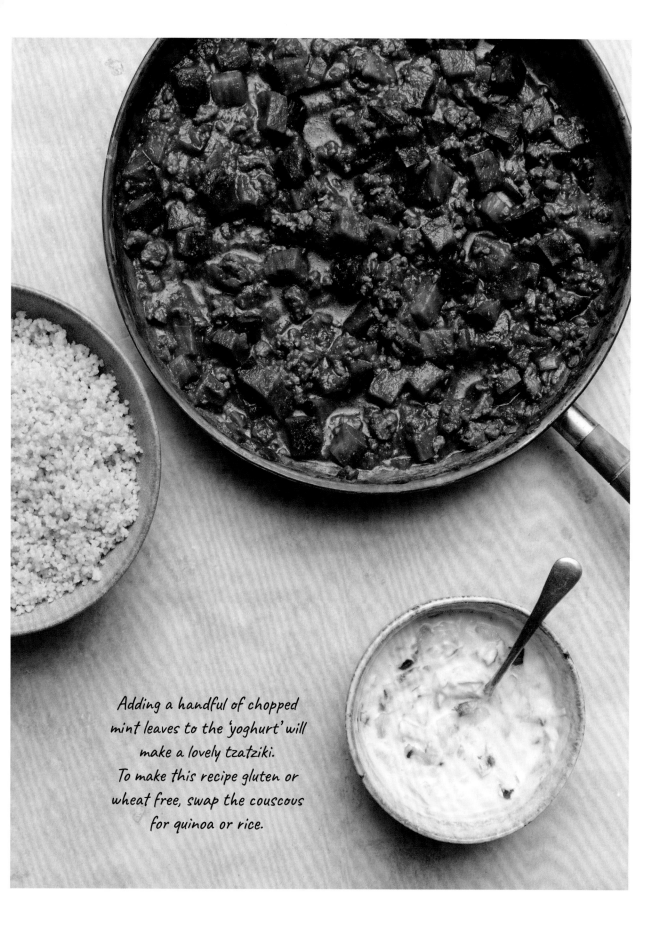

Adding a handful of chopped mint leaves to the 'yoghurt' will make a lovely tzatziki.
To make this recipe gluten or wheat free, swap the couscous for quinoa or rice.

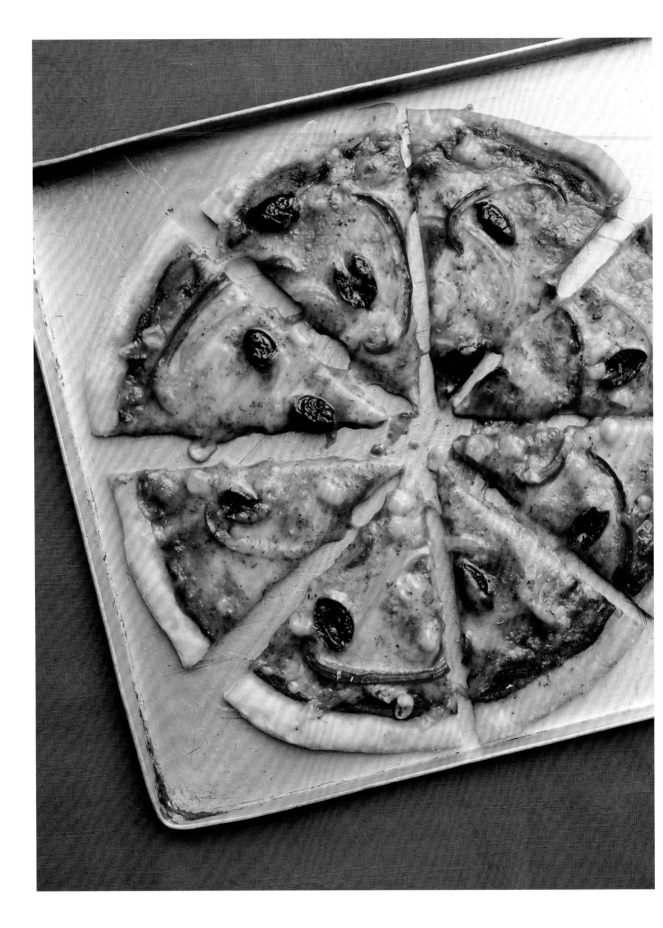

Two-Ingredient Dough Pizza

This dough couldn't be easier to make; as it's yeast-free you don't need to leave it to rest, so the whole meal comes together so quickly. This is a fun one to get your kids involved with making - they'll love picking their toppings and sprinkling over the base!

EF, GF*, NF, PF, SF*, V*, VG*, WF*

Makes: 1 pizza

Prep: 15 minutes, Cook: 15 minutes

toppings of your choice*

60g (2¼oz) Cheddar or mozzarella alternative*

50g (1¾oz) tomato passata

1 tsp tomato purée

½ tsp dried oregano

½ tsp olive oil

FOR THE DOUGH

110g (3¾oz) self-raising flour* (*if using gluten-free flour, add ¼ tsp xanthan gum*)

100g (3½oz) plain Greek-style yoghurt alternative*

1. Preheat the oven to 220°C/Fan 200°C/425°F/Gas Mark 7.

2. Prepare your toppings, including finely grating the cheese alternative.

3. To make your pizza sauce, combine the passata, tomato purée, oregano and olive oil in a small bowl and mix well, then set aside.

4. Next, make your dough. Combine the flour (*plus xanthan gum, if using*) and yoghurt alternative in a large bowl and mix well. Knead with your hands for 5 minutes until combined and resembling dough.

5. Sprinkle some extra flour on to your work surface, then roll out the dough into a thin pizza shape around 23cm (9 in).

6. Spread over the sauce evenly, leaving a small gap around the edges. Sprinkle over the grated cheese alternative, then add the toppings you have chosen.

7. Lift the pizza on to a baking tray lined with baking paper and bake in the oven for 12–15 minutes until the sauce is bubbling.

8. Slice, cool and serve.

STORAGE
Keep covered in the fridge for up to 1 day.

Not suitable for freezing.

Greek-style yoghurt alternative is crucial for this recipe – it won't work well with standard plain yoghurt as you need it to be thick.
Once you've mastered this dough, you can also use it for naan, breadsticks, dough balls, you name it!

Jude's Sausage Pasta

I first posted a version of this recipe a couple of years ago, and it's been so popular that I had to include it here. It's an ideal dinner for when you may have friends of your kids over for tea, as I swear no one would ever know it's dairy free. Named after my little pasta monster Jude because he absolutely loves this dish and has been known to polish off four bowls!

EF, GF*, NF, PF, SF*, WF*

Serves: 2 adults and 2 children

Prep: 10 minutes, Cook: 15 minutes

1 onion

1 garlic clove, peeled

½ courgette

4 sausages* or 200g (7oz) sausage meat*

250g (9oz) pasta*

1 tbsp oil

250g (9oz) tomato passata

125ml (4fl oz) cream alternative*

1 tsp dried oregano

½ tsp yeast extract spread*, such as Marmite® (optional)

1. Dice the onion, garlic and courgette finely.

2. Squeeze out the meat from the sausages (discard the skins) and chop the meat roughly.

3. Cook the pasta according to the packet instructions, reserving a few tablespoons of the starchy cooking water, then drain.

4. Meanwhile, make your sauce. In a large saucepan, heat the oil on a low-medium heat and add the onion, cooking gently for 3 minutes, then add the garlic for a further minute.

5. Add the courgette and cook, stirring often, for a further 2-3 minutes until softening.

6. Turn the heat up to high, add the sausage meat and cook, stirring constantly, for around 3-5 minutes until brown.

7. Add the passata, cream alternative, yeast extract spread (if using) and oregano, stir well, then turn the heat to low and simmer for a few minutes until thickened slightly.

8. Add a couple of tablespoons of the reserved pasta water into the sauce, then pour in the drained pasta, mix together and serve.

STORAGE

Keep covered in the fridge for up to 2 days.

Freeze the sauce for up to 3 months.

Opt for low-salt sausages for young children or replace them with chicken or minced beef or turkey.

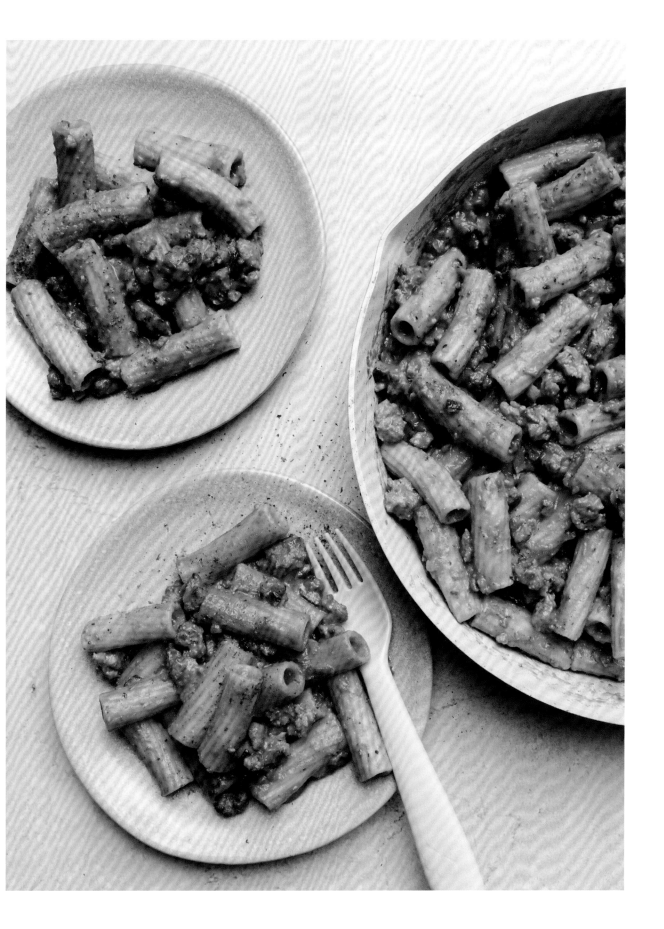

Tuscan-Style Chicken
with Cheat Garlic Bread

The Tuscan-inspired flavours of tomato, smoked paprika and garlic go perfectly with succulent chicken, and how inviting are those vibrant colours? Knock up some cheat garlic bread in a few minutes to dunk, or serve with rice, pasta or potatoes - it's a really versatile dish.

EF, GF*, NF, PF, SF*, WF*

Serves: 2 adults and 2 children

Prep: 10 minutes, Cook: 20 minutes

1 red (bell) pepper

2 garlic cloves, peeled

250g (9oz) cherry tomatoes

150g (5½oz) spinach leaves

500g (1lb 2oz) diced chicken breast

2 tbsp plain flour*

1 tsp ground smoked paprika

1 tsp dried oregano

2 tbsp oil

1 tbsp tomato purée

200ml (7fl oz) hot (low-salt) chicken stock*

150ml (5fl oz) cream alternative*

chopped flat-leaf parsley (optional)

FOR THE CHEAT GARLIC BREAD

sliced baguette or bread*

2 tbsp butter alternative* or margarine*

1 tsp garlic paste

½ tsp dried parsley

1. Prep your veg - dice the red pepper and garlic, cut the tomatoes in half. Wash and roughly chop the spinach leaves.

2. In a bowl, combine the diced chicken, flour, smoked paprika and oregano and mix well so the chicken is all coated.

3. Put a large saucepan on a medium-high heat and add 1½ tablespoons of the oil. When hot, fry the chicken for 6–8 minutes until cooked and golden on all sides, then remove from the pan on to a plate.

4. Add the remaining oil into the pan, then add the pepper, garlic and tomatoes. Cook, stirring often, for 4 minutes until softening.

5. Add the tomato purée and stir for 1 minute, then add the stock and spinach.

6. Bring to the boil, then reduce the heat to low and add the chicken back into the pan, along with the cream alternative. Stir well and simmer for a few minutes until the chicken is cooked through.

7. Meanwhile, make your cheat garlic bread. Pop the slices of baguette or bread into the toaster until lightly toasted. Mix the butter alternative or margarine in a bowl, stir in the garlic paste and dried parsley and cook in the microwave for 30 seconds until melted. Spread on to the toasted bread slices.

8. Serve the chicken, scattered with chopped flat-leaf parsley if you wish, with the cheat garlic bread on the side.

STORAGE
Keep covered in the fridge for up to 2 days.

Freeze sauce for up to 3 months.

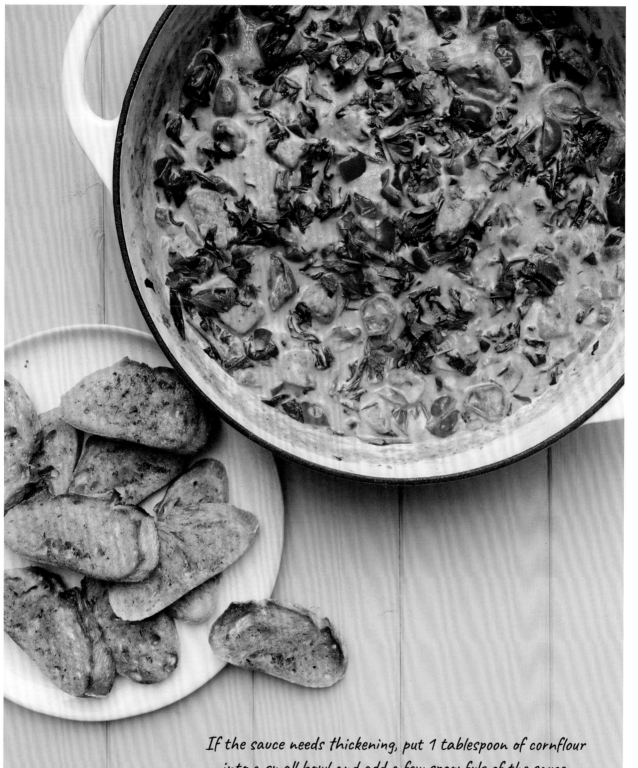

If the sauce needs thickening, put 1 tablespoon of cornflour into a small bowl and add a few spoonfuls of the sauce. Stir well to form a paste, then add back into the pan and stir through thoroughly.

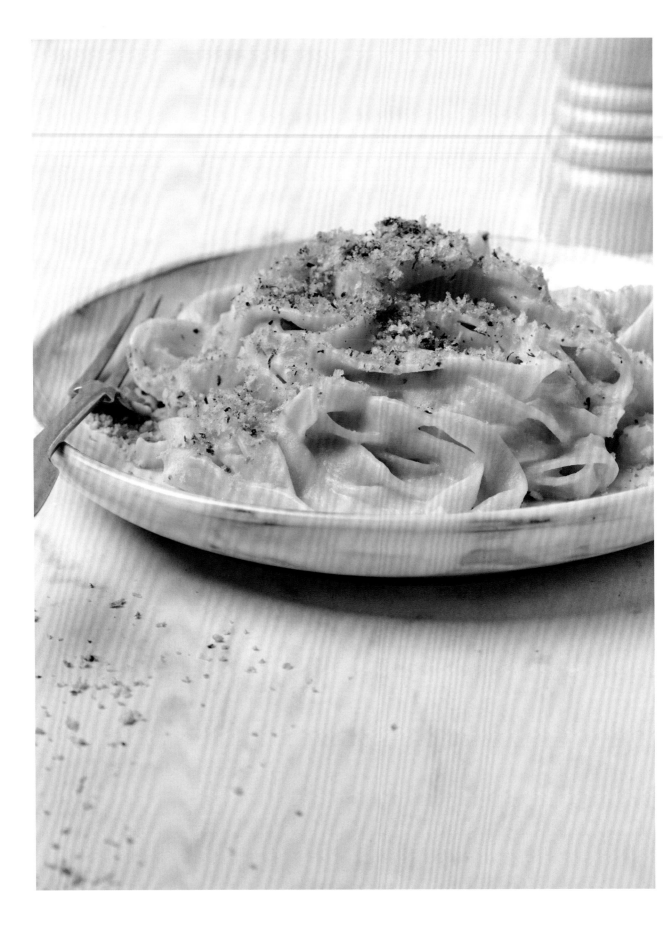

Cauliflower Alfredo

Alfredo is typically a combination of butter, cream and cheese, so basically full of dairy! Here's a twist everyone can enjoy - a comforting, creamy sauce made from nutritious cauliflower, with a herb breadcrumb topping. Ideal with tagliatelle, or the pasta of your choice.

EF, GF*, NF, PF, SF*, V, VG, WF*

Serves: 2 adults and 2 children

Prep: 10-15 minutes, Cook: 15 minutes

1 cauliflower, florets only (approx. 450g/1lb)

1 onion

3 garlic cloves, peeled

1 tbsp butter alternative* or margarine*

250ml (9fl oz) hot (low-salt) vegetable stock*

200ml (7fl oz) plant-based milk alternative*

4 tbsp nutritional yeast

300g (10½ oz) tagliatelle*

FOR THE HERB BREADCRUMBS

1 tsp butter alternative* or margarine*

2 tbsp panko breadcrumbs*, (or gluten-free breadcrumbs)

½ tsp dried mixed herbs

1. Chop the cauliflower florets into chunks, discarding any green leaves. Dice the onion and garlic.

2. In a large saucepan, heat the butter alternative or margarine on a medium heat, then add the onion and garlic and cook for 3 minutes until softening.

3. Add the cauliflower, hot stock and milk alternative. Bring to the boil, then simmer for 10-12 minutes until the cauliflower is soft.

4. Add the contents of the pan to a blender, along with the nutritional yeast and blend.

5. Meanwhile, cook your pasta according to the packet instructions.

6. To make the herb breadcrumbs, melt the butter alternative or margarine in a small pan on a medium heat, then add the panko breadcrumbs and herbs. Stir to coat the breadcrumbs in the butter alternative and toast, stirring often, until golden. Tip on to a plate and leave to cool.

7. Combine the drained pasta with the sauce, mix well and heat through, then serve topped with the herb breadcrumbs.

STORAGE
Keep covered in the fridge for up to 3 days.

The sauce can be frozen (without breadcrumbs) for up to 3 months.

If you're not a fan of cauliflower, this method will also work with sweet potato or butternut squash - just make sure they're soft before blending.

Snacks & On-The-Go

Tasty and nutritious options are so helpful to have on hand when you get those inevitable snack requests! These recipes are designed to work for whatever stage your family is at. They make excellent finger food for weaning, are ideal to pack in a lunchbox, or as snacks between meals or after school. I like to load up the freezer with the freezable ones and defrost a batch regularly to have on hand for the week ahead.

No-Bake Bliss Balls

So easy to whip up, these delicious bites are packed with energy-boosting ingredients, as well as protein, calcium and iron.

EF, GF*, PF*, SF, V, VG, WF*

Makes: 6

Prep: 15 minutes, Chill: 30 minutes

1 small banana

50g (1¾oz) porridge oats*

1 tbsp smooth nut butter*

1 tbsp chia seeds

2 tbsp plain Greek-style yoghurt alternative*

4 tbsp desiccated coconut

1. In a large bowl, mash the banana, then add the oats, nut butter, chia seeds and yoghurt alternative and mix well.

2. Refrigerate for 5 minutes (this makes them easier to roll).

3. Pour the desiccated coconut on to a plate.

4. Divide the mix into 6 pieces and roll each one into a ball, then roll in the coconut until coated all over.

5. Pop into the fridge for 30 minutes to firm up before eating.

STORAGE
Keep covered in the fridge for up to 1 day.

Not suitable for freezing.

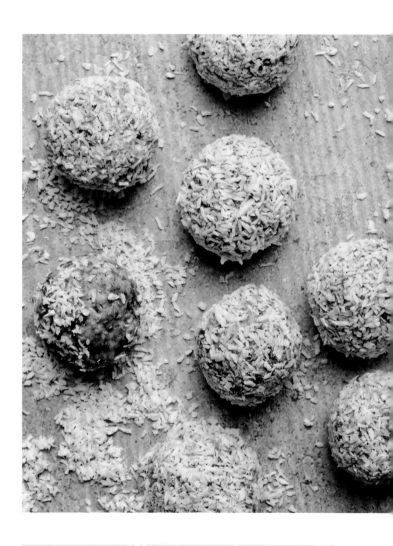

Add some crumbled frozen raspberries for a fruity twist.

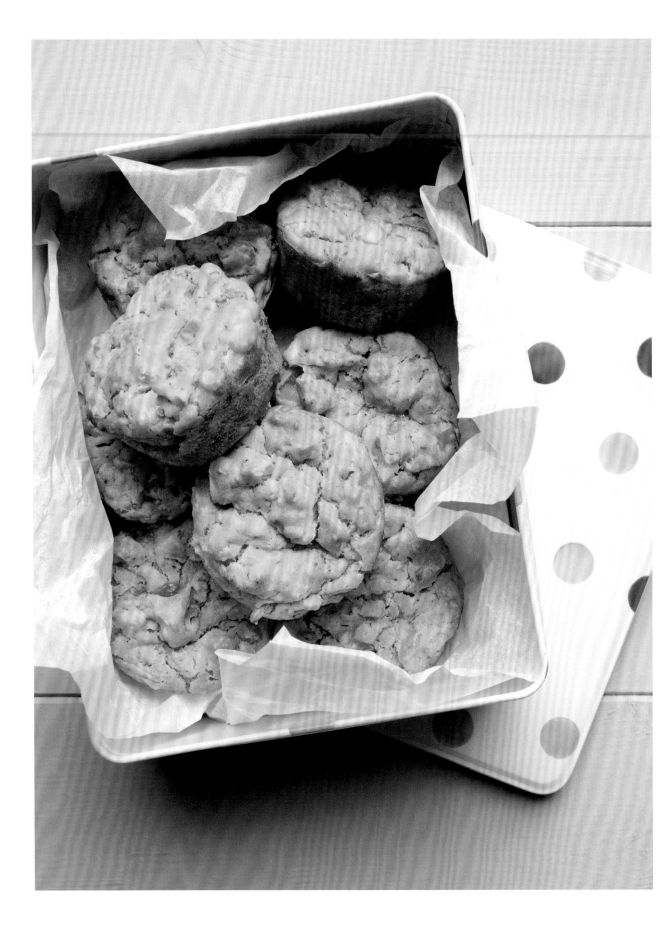

Carrot & Corn Savoury Muffins

Savoury muffins are an excellent choice for lunchboxes, and these ones are fluffy, tasty and nutritious. Try cutting in half and toasting, then spreading dairy-free butter on top – delicious!

GF*, NF, PF, SF*, V, WF*

Makes: 12

Prep: 15 minutes, Cook: 20–22 minutes

2 medium carrots (approx. 220g/8oz)

1 large egg

250ml (9fl oz) plant-based milk alternative*

250g (9oz) self-raising flour* (*if using gluten-free flour, add ¼ tsp xanthan gum*)

1 tsp baking powder

100g (3½oz) Cheddar alternative*

50ml (2fl oz) light vegetable oil, plus extra for greasing

150g (5½oz) canned sweetcorn

1 tsp dried mixed herbs

1. Preheat the oven to 190°C/Fan 170°C/375°F/Gas Mark 5 and grease a 12-hole muffin tin.

2. Peel and grate the carrots.

3. In a large bowl, beat the egg, then add the milk alternative and mix well.

4. In a separate bowl, mix together the flour (*plus xanthan gum, if using*), baking powder and grate in the Cheddar alternative.

5. Add the oil, grated carrot, sweetcorn and dried herbs.

6. Pour in the egg and milk alternative mixture, then mix and fold everything together to combine.

7. Divide the mix evenly between the muffin holes.

8. Bake for 20–22 minutes until a knife comes out clean, then cool in the tin for 10 minutes and remove on to a wire rack to cool completely.

STORAGE
Keep covered in the fridge for up to 3 days.

Freeze for up to 3 months.

If egg free, you can replace the egg with a chia or flax seed egg (see page 76).

Tropical Oat Bars

Gorgeous, tropical flavours of mango, banana and coconut in soft oaty fingers.
With slow releasing energy, these make an ideal snack, or a lovely breakfast.

EF, GF*, NF, PF, SF, V, VG, WF*

Makes: 12

Prep: 5–10 minutes, Cook: 25–30 minutes

1 mango

80g (2¾oz) coconut oil, plus extra for greasing

180g (6oz) porridge oats*

2 tbsp desiccated coconut

2 ripe bananas

1. Preheat the oven to 190°C/Fan 170°C/375°F/Gas Mark 5 and line or grease a 20cm (8in) square baking tin.

2. Peel and chop the mango into small pieces – if it is very ripe, blot any excess liquid from the fruit with a piece of kitchen paper.

3. Melt the coconut oil in a small pan over a low heat and add to a bowl with the mango, porridge oats and desiccated coconut.

4. Mash the bananas and add to the bowl, then give everything a good mix.

5. Pour the mix into the prepared baking tin and ensure it is evenly spread, then press down firmly all over to compact the mix.

6. Bake for 25–30 minutes until golden.

7. Leave to cool completely in the tin, then slice into 12 bars.

STORAGE
Keep covered in the fridge for up to 3 days.

Freeze for up to 3 months.

For a coconut-free alternative, use vegetable oil and replace the desiccated coconut with ground almonds or omit completely.

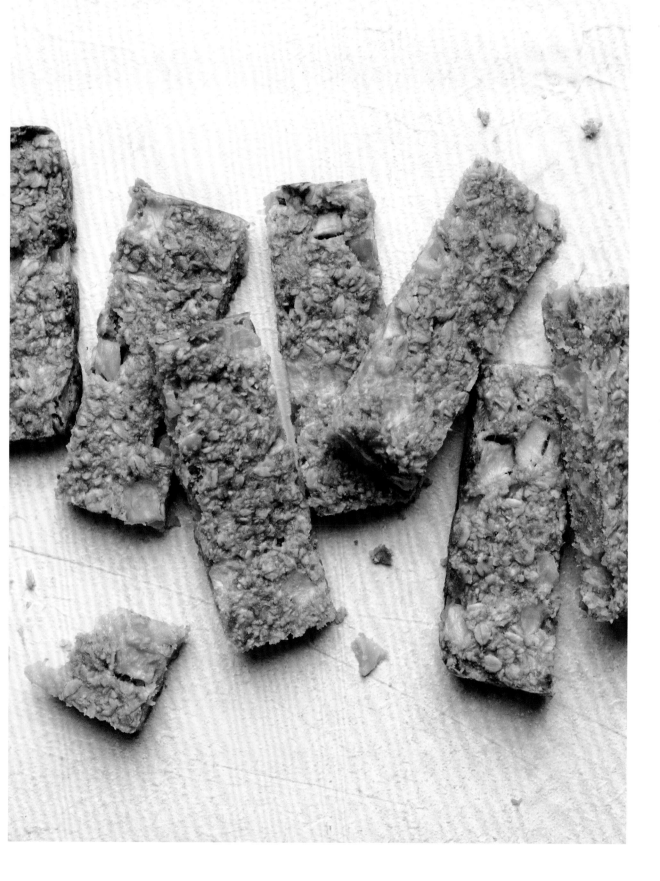

PBJ Twists

The classic flavours of peanut butter and jam in a flaky pastry twist. Simple but impressive, these would also be great for a playdate or party.

EF*, GF*, NF*, SF*, V*, VG*, WF*

Makes: 20

Prep: 20 minutes, Cook: 10–12 minutes

320g (11½oz) pack of ready-rolled puff pastry*

2 tbsp smooth peanut butter

2 tbsp low-sugar jam (or Strawberry Chia Jam, see page 86)

beaten egg* or plant-based milk alternative*, for glazing

1. Preheat the oven to 220°C/Fan 200°C /425°F/Gas Mark 7, and line two large baking trays with baking paper. Remove the pastry from the fridge 10 minutes before use.

2. Unroll the pastry so it's landscape, then – imagining there's a line down the middle – spread the peanut butter over one half, and the jam over the other half.

3. Fold one side over the other, left to right (like a book!). Then, using a pizza cutter or sharp knife, cut into 10 strips from the top down.

4. Take each strip, cut it in half to make them half the length, then brush all over with the beaten egg or milk alternative. You should have 20 short strips.

5. Holding the strip at either end, twist in opposite directions until it resembles a spiral.

6. Put on to the prepared baking trays and repeat for all strips, leaving a 2.5cm (1in) gap between each twist.

7. Bake for 10–12 minutes until crispy and golden.

STORAGE
Keep covered in the fridge for up to 2 days.

Not suitable for freezing.

If peanut free, you could swap for another nut butter, or use jam on both sides.

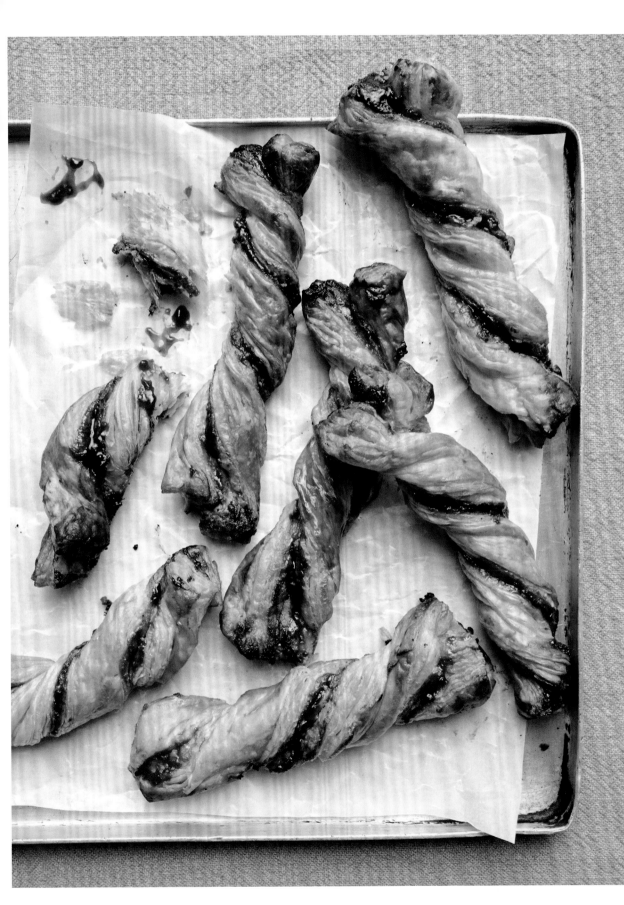

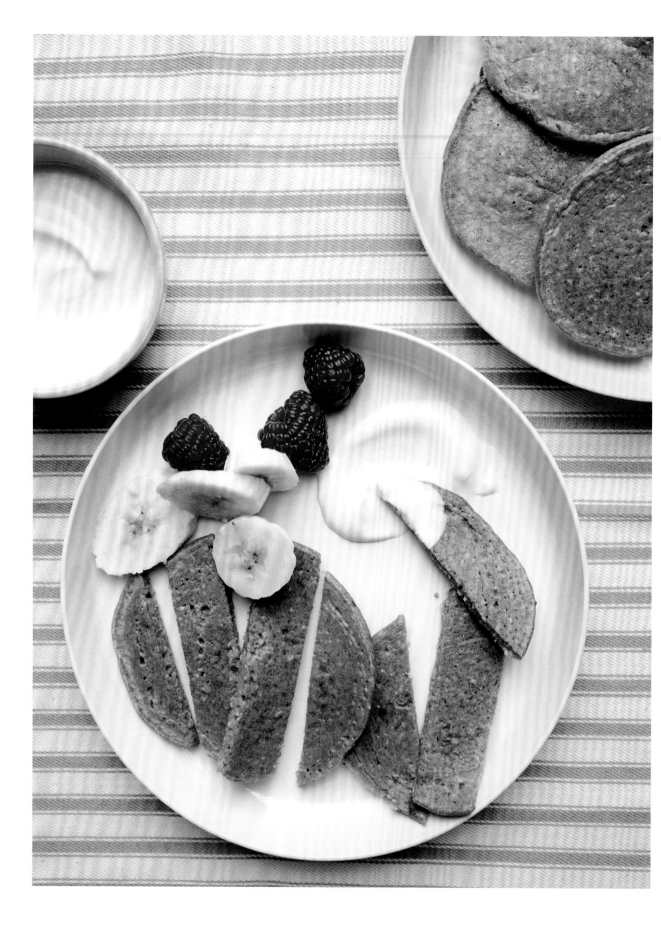

Spinach & Banana Pancakes

Full of green goodness, with the natural sweetness of banana. These are a great texture for weaning, but then call them 'hulk pancakes' and watch the older kids dive in too...

EF, GF* NF, PF, SF*, V, VG, WF*

Makes: 18

Prep: 10 minutes, Cook: 10 minutes

50g (1¾oz) spinach leaves

1 banana

130g (4½oz) porridge oats*

60g (2¼oz) plain flour*

250ml (9fl oz) plant-based milk alternative*

oil

1. Wash the spinach, then add to a blender with the banana, porridge oats, flour and milk alternative. Blend well.

2. Drizzle a little oil into a non-stick frying pan on a medium heat.

3. Add 1 tablespoon of pancake mixture per pancake, flatten with the spoon into a pancake shape and cook for 1-2 minutes on each side, flipping when it's starting to colour. You will need to do this in batches until the mixture is used up.

4. Cool, and serve.

STORAGE
Keep covered in the fridge for up to 3 days.

Freeze for up to 3 months.

For an extra nutritional boost, add 1 tablespoon of milled chia or flax seeds when blending the ingredients.

Salmon & Potato Croquettes
with a Lemon & Herb Dip

Canned salmon is an excellent source of calcium, protein and omega-3 fats. These crispy croquettes are delicious - next time you're making a meal with mashed potatoes, make some extra and give these a try.

EF, GF*, NF, PF, SF*, WF*

Makes: 12

Prep: 10 minutes, Cook: 25 minutes

300g (10½oz) potatoes

105g (3¾oz) can salmon

1 tsp chopped fresh or dried parsley

40g (1½oz) panko breadcrumbs* (or gluten-free breadcrumbs)

oil

FOR THE LEMON & HERB DIP

3 tbsp plain Greek-style yoghurt alternative*

1 tbsp flat-leaf parsley, finely chopped

zest of ½ lemon

1. Peel and chop the potatoes, add to a large saucepan of boiling water and cook for 15 minutes. Drain, mash well and leave to cool.

2. Open the can of salmon, drain, and remove and discard any skin.

3. Add the salmon to the mashed potatoes along with the parsley and mash together until all combined.

4. Put the breadcrumbs on a plate. Using damp hands, take 1 heaped teaspoon of the mixture, roll into a ball, then shape into a croquette. Press into the breadcrumbs until coated on all sides. Repeat until you have 12 croquettes.

5. In a non-stick frying pan, heat 1 tablespoon of oil on a medium-high heat and fry the croquettes for 2 minutes on each side until crispy and golden.

6. Repeat, adding more oil when the pan is looking dry.

7. In a small bowl, mix together all the ingredients for the lemon and herb dip.

8. Serve the croquettes with the lemon and herb dip on the side.

STORAGE
Keep covered in the fridge for up to 2 days.

Freeze for up to 3 months.

As well as making a healthy snack, you could also serve these as a main meal with veggies.

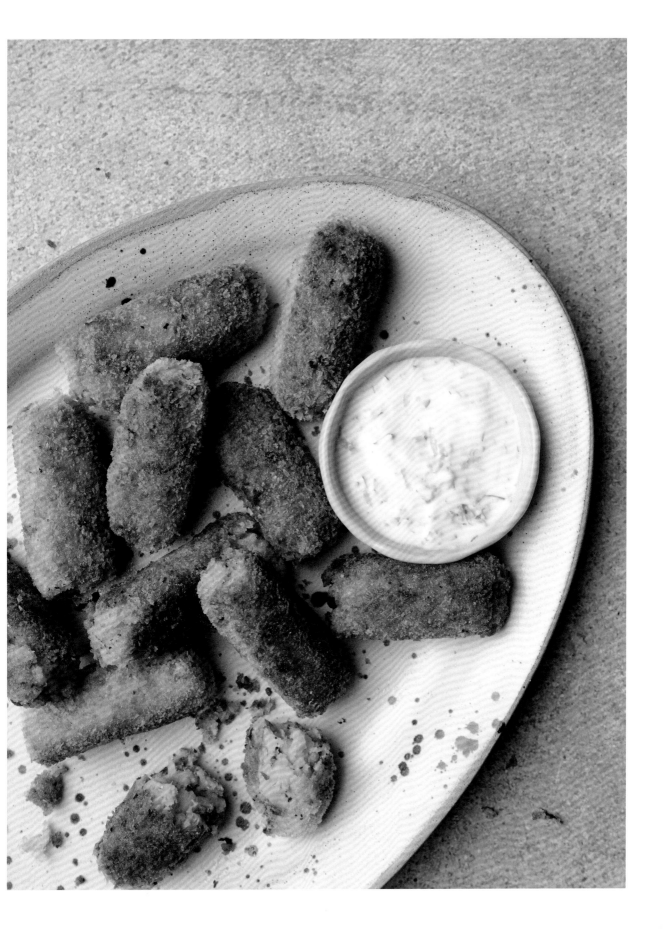

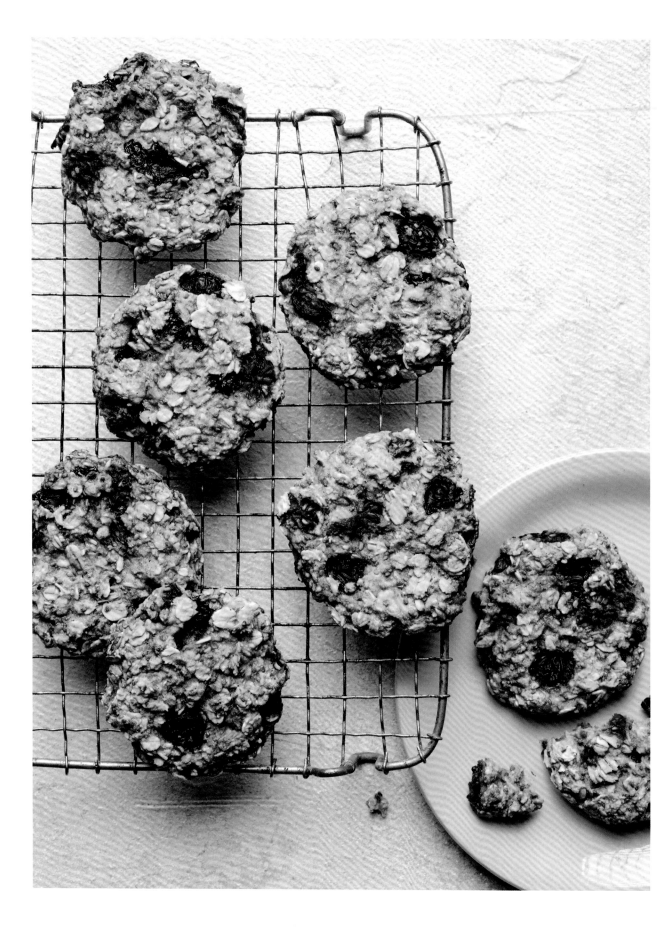

Berry & Chia Seed Cookies

These oat cookies are one of my most popular allergy-friendly recipes ever. They're squidgy, so a suitable texture for all ages and my kids absolutely love them. I'm also partial to one with my afternoon coffee!

EF, GF*, NF, PF, SF, V, VG, WF*

Makes: 8

Prep: 10 minutes, Cook: 20–22 minutes

2 ripe bananas

90g (3¼oz) porridge oats*

1 tbsp chia seeds

80g (2¾oz) fresh or frozen berries

1. Preheat the oven to 200°C/Fan 180°C/400°F/Gas Mark 6 and line a baking tray with baking paper.

2. Mash the bananas in a large bowl until smooth, then add the oats and chia seeds and stir well.

3. Chop the berries into small pieces and add to the bowl, then fold into the mixture.

4. Shape into 8 thick cookies and place on the prepared baking tray.

5. Bake for 20–22 minutes until golden around the edges.

6. Leave to cool on the tray for a few minutes before transferring them to a wire rack to cool completely.

STORAGE
Keep covered in the fridge for up to 3 days.

Freeze for up to 3 months.

The browner the bananas you use, the sweeter the cookies!
This basic recipe is really versatile – you can also try different fruit or adding nut butter.

Lentil & Courgette Fritters

Fritters are a popular baby-led weaning dish, but they also make a tasty snack for the whole family. Mildly spiced and packed with plant-based protein and iron, these would work really well with my Cucumber 'Yoghurt' Dip (see page 152).

EF, NF, PF, SF, V, VG

Makes: 12

Prep: 15 minutes, Cook: 15 minutes

100g (3½oz) split red lentils

200g (7oz) courgette

60g (2¼oz) plain flour

1 tsp ground cumin

1 tsp dried parsley

oil

1. Rinse the lentils in a sieve under cold water for 2 minutes, then cook in a saucepan of boiling water for 10 minutes until just tender. Drain well.

2. Meanwhile, grate the courgette and squeeze out any excess liquid using a clean tea towel.

3. Add the courgette and drained lentils to a bowl, then add the flour, cumin and parsley and mix well. Shape into 12 fritters.

4. In a non-stick frying pan, heat 1 tablespoon of oil on a medium heat and cook the fritters in batches for 3-4 minutes on each side until golden. Remove from the pan on to kitchen paper to absorb any excess oil. Repeat until all the fritters are cooked, then cool and serve.

STORAGE
Keep covered in the fridge for up to 3 days.

Freeze for up to 3 months.

When you drain the lentils, squash them down into the sieve with a spoon to get rid of all the water; this will result in crispier fritters.

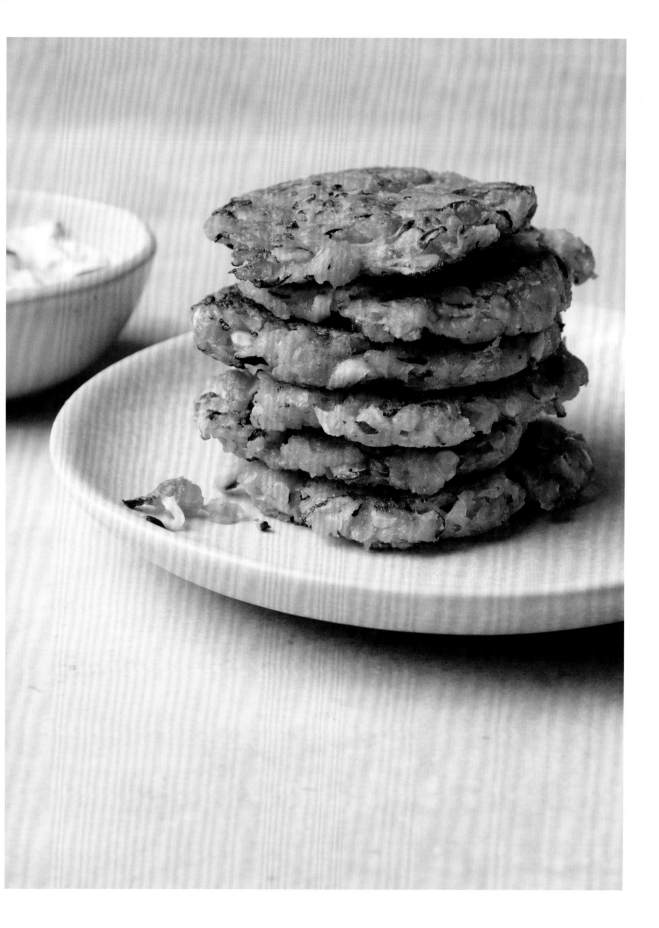

Puddings & Sweet Treats

If you've ever stared longingly at the dessert fridge in the supermarket, packed full of dairy-laden treats you can't have, I've got your back. No one should miss out on a good pud – all of these recipes are also egg free.

There's a range from healthy options to more decadent treats here – each is marked as 'suitable for' either all ages, 1 year + or older kids and adults, depending on the sugar content.

5-Minute Cookie Mug Cake

Cookie dough meets fluffy cake in this super-easy mug cake made in the microwave. This is perfect when you need a quick sweet fix, as it's ready in just five minutes from start to finish. Add some dairy-free whipped cream or ice cream for ultimate luxury.

EF, GF*, NF, PF, SF*, V, VG, WF*

Serves: 1

Prep: 4 minutes, Cook: 1 minute

Suitable for: older kids and adults

1 tbsp plant-based milk alternative*

¼ tsp vanilla extract

1 tbsp oil

1 tbsp coconut sugar (or brown sugar)

3 tbsp self-raising flour*

10g (¼oz) dairy-free chocolate chips or chunks*

1. In a small microwave-safe mug or ramekin, add the plant-based milk alternative, vanilla extract, oil and sugar, and stir well to mix.

2. Add the flour and mix again until all combined.

3. Fold in the chocolate chips or chunks and sprinkle a few on top.

4. Microwave on high for 1 minute, then leave to cool for a minute and serve.

STORAGE
Best served fresh.

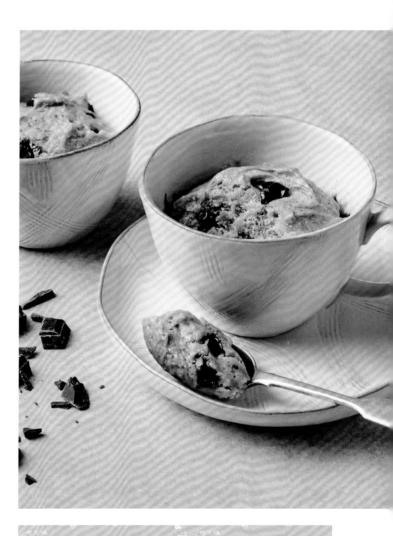

If using coconut oil, ensure it is melted before you begin the recipe.

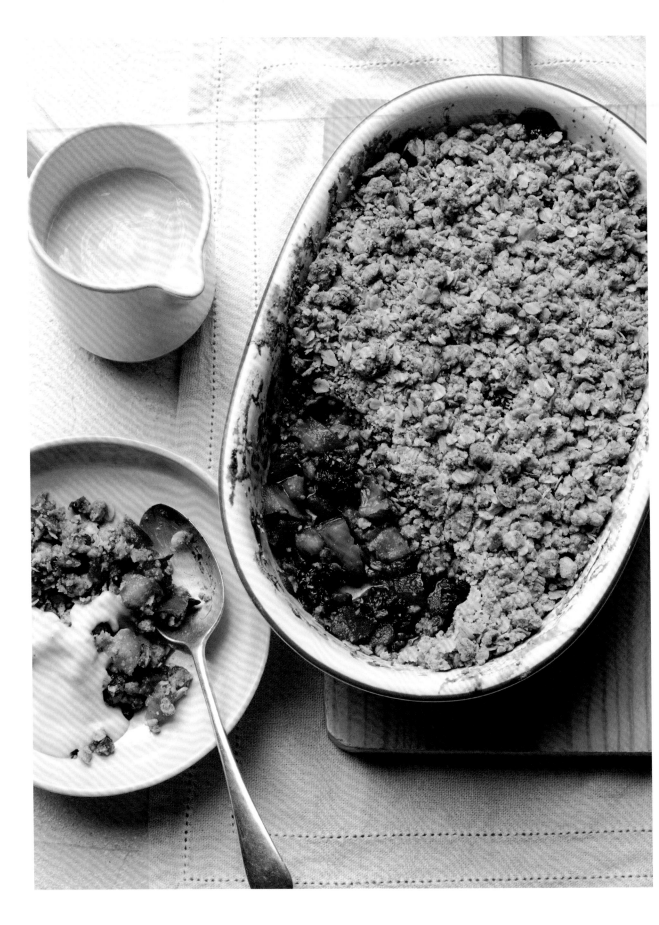

Pear & Blackberry Crumble

Juicy blackberries and sweet pear combine beautifully with a crunchy, granola-style topping. A good crumble is hard to beat, and this reduced sugar version is our favourite family dessert. Now the only question that remains is: are you team custard or ice cream? Dairy free, of course!

EF, GF*, NF, PF, SF*, V, VG, WF*

Serves: 2 adults and 2 children

Prep: 15 minutes, Cook: 40 minutes

Suitable for: 1 year+

FOR THE FILLING

3 ripe pears (approx. 380g/13½oz)

150g (5½oz) fresh or frozen blackberries

1 tbsp lemon juice

1 tbsp coconut sugar (or light brown sugar)

1 tsp vanilla extract

FOR THE TOPPING

100g (3½oz) plain flour*

80g (2¾oz) porridge or rolled oats*

90g (3¼oz) butter alternative* or margarine*, plus (optional) extra for greasing

2 tbsp coconut sugar (or light brown sugar)

1 tsp ground cinnamon

1. Preheat the oven to 200°C/Fan 180°C/400°F/Gas Mark 6 and grease a 23cm x 14cm (9 x 5½ inch) oval or rectangular baking dish.

2. To make the filling, chop the pears into chunks, discarding the core. Cut the blackberries in half. Add to a bowl with the lemon juice and sugar, stir well to mix, then pour into the prepared baking dish.

3. Now make your topping. Add all the ingredients to a large bowl and mix together with your hands, rubbing together with your fingers until it looks like granola.

4. Spread the topping evenly over the fruit mix.

5. Bake for 40 minutes until golden and bubbling. Cool and serve.

STORAGE
Keep covered in the fridge for up to 3 days.

Freeze for up to 3 months.

I like using coconut sugar for this, as it gives a slightly caramel taste, but brown sugar will work just as well.

Banana & Strawberry 'Nice Cream'

Just three ingredients is all it takes to make this tasty, refreshing ice cream alternative. The natural sweetness of the fruit means there's no need for sugar, so it's baby-friendly and also great for teething, illness or a heatwave!

EF, GF*, NF, PF, SF*, V, VG, WF*

Serves: 2 adults and 2 children

Prep: 10 minutes, Chill: 4+ hours

Suitable for: all ages

2 bananas

200g (7oz) fresh or frozen strawberries

90ml (6 tbsp) plant-based milk alternative*

1. Chop the bananas into chunks, remove the stalks from the strawberries and cut them in half.

2. Place in a lidded storage container and put in the freezer overnight, or for a minimum of 4 hours.

3. Add the frozen fruit to a food processor or high-speed blender with the milk alternative, pulse a few times, then blend until it's the consistency of soft-serve ice cream.

4. Serve straight away or refreeze for 1 hour.

STORAGE
Freeze for up to 6 months.

Bananas are needed to give the creamy consistency, but you can experiment with different fruits to pair with them – cherries and peach are two of our favourites. Get the kids involved by offering them toppings to add themselves – it could be loosened peanut butter, desiccated coconut or sugar sprinkles for older children.

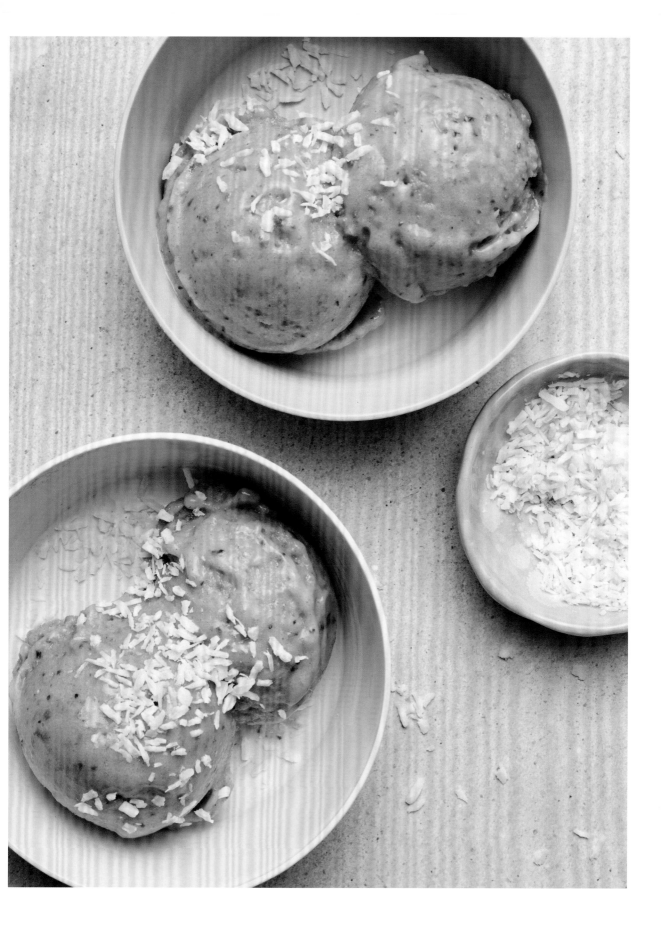

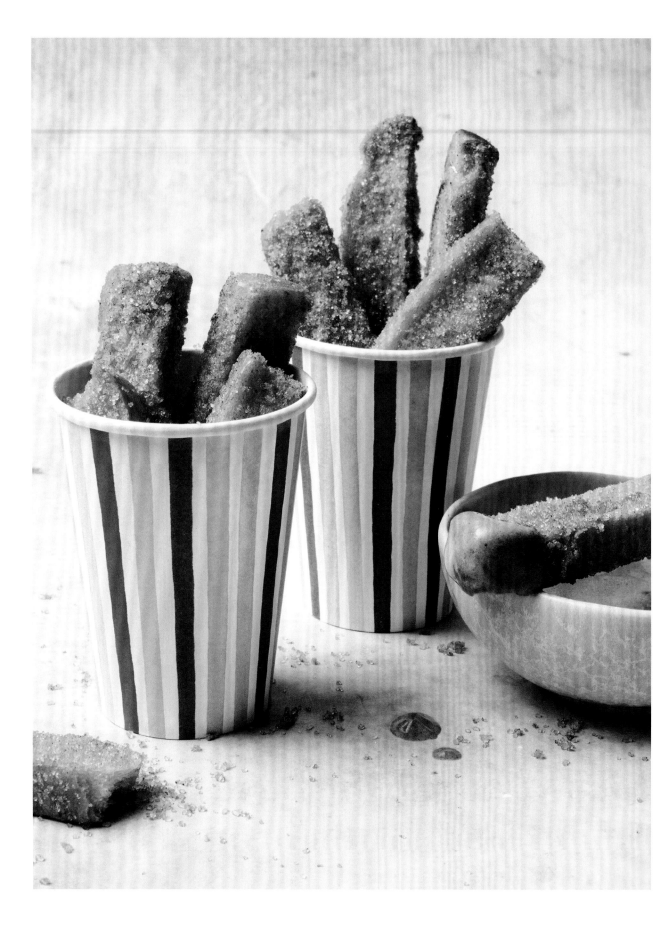

Bread Crust 'Churros'
with a Choc 'Yoghurt' Dip

Anyone else with kids always end up throwing loads of bread crusts away? Well, save them and give these delicious cinnamon sugar 'churros' a go... Be warned though, they're seriously moreish!

EF, GF*, NF, PF, SF*, V, VG, WF*

Makes: 8

Prep: 10 minutes, Cook: 10 minutes

Suitable for: older kids and adults

½ tsp ground cinnamon

2 tbsp demerara sugar

2 tbsp butter alternative* or margarine*

2 slices of bread*, crusts only

FOR THE CHOC 'YOGHURT' DIP

120g (4¼oz) plain Greek-style yoghurt alternative*

1 tsp cocoa powder

1 tsp maple syrup

1. Preheat the oven to 200°C/Fan 180°C/400°F/Gas Mark 6 and line a baking tray with baking paper.

2. On a plate, mix together the cinnamon and sugar.

3. Melt the butter alternative or margarine in the microwave or in a saucepan.

4. Dip each bread crust into the melted butter alternative or margarine so it's coated all over, then roll in the cinnamon sugar mix.

5. Place on the baking tray and repeat the process. Bake for 8-10 minutes, turning halfway through cooking until golden and crispy.

6. Meanwhile, make the dip by combining all the ingredients in a small bowl.

7. Cool and serve the 'churros' with the dip on the side.

STORAGE
Best served fresh.

Stale bread works best for these – I like tiger bread for a nice thick crust.
To make these suitable for smaller children, you could roll in desiccated coconut instead of the cinnamon sugar mix.

Mini No-Bake 'Cheesecakes'

Cheesecake might be a dessert you'll think is off the menu when you're dairy free, but fear not with these delightful mini ones! Crunchy biscuit bases with a light, creamy topping and decorated with the fruit of your choice.

EF, GF*, NF, PF, SF*, V, VG, WF*

Makes: 12

Prep: 20 minutes, Chill: 6+ hours

Suitable for: 1 year+

FOR THE BASE

125g (4½oz) dairy-free digestive-style biscuits*

50g (1¾oz) butter alternative* or margarine*

FOR THE TOPPING

100ml (3½fl oz) whippable double cream alternative*

150g (5½oz) soft cheese alternative*

3 tbsp maple syrup

2 tbsp plain Greek-style yoghurt alternative*

½ tsp lemon juice

2 tsp vanilla extract

fruit of choice, to decorate

1. Start by making the bases. Place the biscuits in a large bowl and bash with a rolling pin until all crumbled. Melt the butter alternative or margarine and add, then mix together well until combined.

2. Line a 12-hole muffin tin with cupcake cases and distribute the biscuit base evenly between them. Press each base down with a spoon until compacted. Put the tin in the fridge while you make the filling.

3. Whip the cream alternative until it forms stiff peaks.

4. In a separate bowl, add the soft cheese alternative, maple syrup, yoghurt alternative, lemon juice and vanilla extract, then mix well.

5. Fold in the whipped cream alternative gently.

6. Take the tin out of the fridge and spoon over the topping, making sure it's evenly divided. Cover the tin and pop back in the fridge overnight to set (or for 6 hours minimum).

7. When ready to serve, remove from the cupcake cases and decorate with berries, sliced banana or chopped mango or peach.

STORAGE
Keep covered in the fridge for up to 2 days.

Freeze for up to 3 months, then defrost in the fridge.

Ensure you use cupcake cases to line your tin to maker it easier to remove the cheesecakes once chilled.

Make sure you check the ingredients on the digestive biscuits, as some brands contain milk!

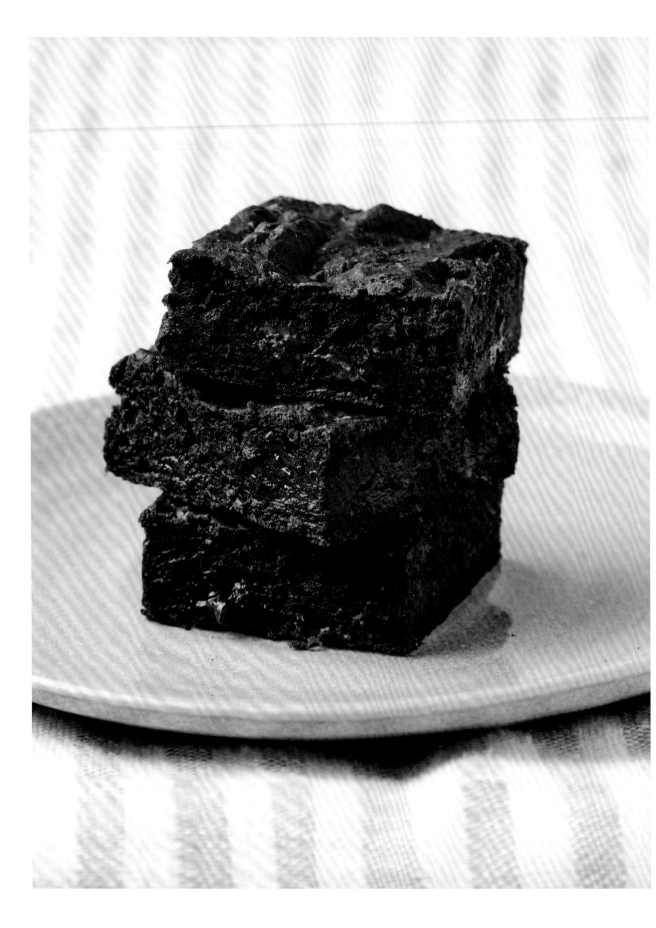

Squidgy Black Bean Brownies

No one will guess the secret ingredient to these brownies is a can of calcium and iron-rich black beans! Fudgy, sweet and delicious - these need to be tasted to be believed.

EF, GF*, NF, PF, SF*, V, VG, WF*

Makes: 16

Prep: 20 minutes, Cook: 22–25 minutes

Suitable for: 1 year+

2 tbsp chia seeds

400g (14oz) can black beans

75ml (2½fl oz) maple syrup

3 tsp vanilla extract

75ml (2½fl oz) oil, plus (optional) extra for greasing

75ml (2½fl oz) plant-based milk alternative*

75g (2½oz) plain flour*

3 tbsp cocoa powder

1 tsp baking powder

¼ tsp bicarbonate of soda

100g (3½oz) dairy-free chocolate chips or chunks*

1. Preheat the oven to 200°C/Fan 180°C/400°F/Gas Mark 6 and line or grease a 20cm (8in) square baking tin.

2. Put the chia seeds in a small bowl and cover with 5 tablespoons of cold water, stir well, then leave for 15 minutes until gel-like in texture (this is your chia egg).

3. Meanwhile, drain and rinse the black beans and add to a food processor, along with the maple syrup, vanilla extract, oil and milk alternative. Pulse until the beans are chopped up.

4. Add the flour, cocoa powder, baking powder and bicarbonate of soda, then blend until smooth, scraping down the sides of the blender bowl with a spatula to ensure it's all mixed.

5. Add the chia egg and blend again for 10 seconds.

6. Gently fold in the chocolate chips or chunks, then pour the mixture into the prepared baking tin and spread evenly.

7. Bake for 22–25 minutes until crusty on top and springy to the touch (less cooking time will result in a fudgier texture).

8. Cool in the tin for at least 20 minutes, then cut into 16 pieces.

STORAGE
Keep covered in the fridge for up to 3 days.

Freeze for up to 6 months.

Serve warm to adults and/or bigger kids portions with a scoop of dairy-free ice cream.

Fruit Pizza

This is a really quick, easy and fun idea for kids, which also happens to be nutritious! All the toppings are fruit based, with jam for 'pizza sauce', mashed banana for 'cheese', watermelon for 'pepperoni' and blueberries for 'olives'.

EF, GF*, NF, PF, SF*, V, VG, WF*

Serves: 1

Prep: 5–10 minutes

Suitable for: all ages

1 slice of bread*

½ ripe banana

fruit 'toppings' (see intro)

low-sugar or Strawberry Chia Jam (see page 86)

1. Toast the bread, mash the banana and slice the toppings.

2. Cut the toast in half diagonally. Spread the jam over the toast in a thin layer, then top with the mashed banana and decorate with the fruit toppings.

STORAGE
Best served fresh.

Why not get the kids involved with choosing and cutting the toppings? Or even have a contest to see who can make the best pizza!

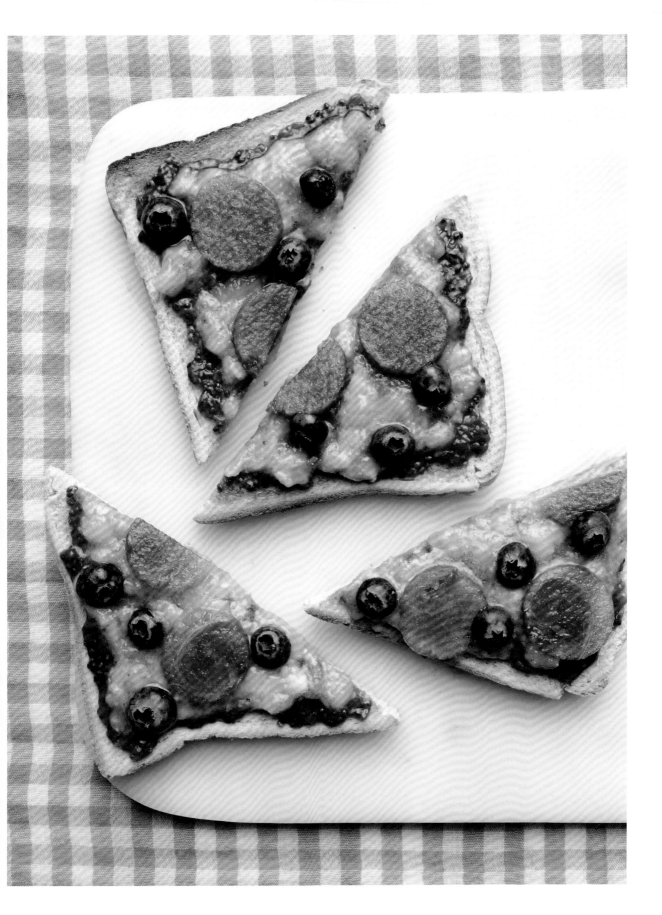

Party Food

For me, parties and celebrations should be about total joy and indulgence, seeing everyone with happy faces and full bellies. For allergy parents, it also means a lot for your child to feel included, eating the same food as everyone else, and getting to enjoy yummy treats.

Here's a selection of recipes for your special occasion. There's no age guideline on these because I'm a firm believer in that when it comes to parties, even babies can have a little taste of the cake!

Cutie Fruity Kebabs

A really fun and inviting way to serve fruit at a party. Grab some cutter shapes, choose lots of different coloured fruit, then get creative with your designs!

EF, GF, NF, PF, SF, V, VG, WF

Prep: 10-15 minutes

fruit of choice (I use melon, pineapple, mango and blueberries)

wooden skewers

1. Cut your fruit into different shapes using cutters.

2. Thread a large shape on the top of a wooden skewer, then fill below it with more fruit shapes and berries.

STORAGE
Best served fresh.

Make sure you snip the sharp edges off the skewers, and that any small round fruit like grapes and blueberries are cut in half if serving to young children.

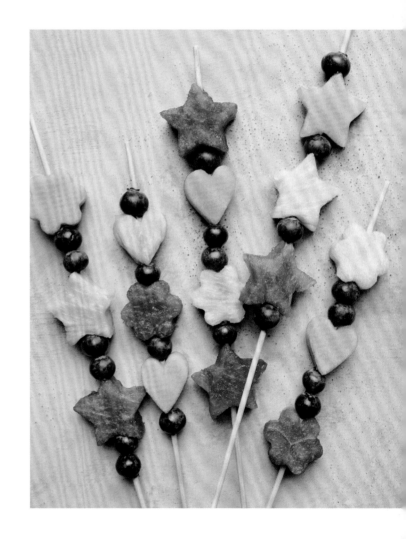

Pizza Pinwheels

I have fond memories of my mum teaching me to make a version of these when I was young and just starting to get interested in cooking. What's brilliant about these is they're so simple to prepare but are loved by all ages - you can't go wrong with a pinwheel.

EF*, GF*, NF, PF, SF*, V, VG, WF*

Makes: 18-20

Prep: 20 minutes, Cook: 20 minutes

320g (11½oz) pack of ready-rolled puff pastry*

65g (2¼oz) Cheddar alternative*

2 tbsp tomato purée

1 tsp dried mixed herbs

beaten egg* or plant-based milk alternative*, for glazing

1. Preheat the oven to 200°C/Fan 180°C /400°F/Gas Mark 6 and line two baking trays with baking paper.

2. Take the pastry out of the fridge for 10 minutes before unrolling.

3. Meanwhile, grate your Cheddar alternative finely and make your sauce by adding 3 tablespoons of water to the tomato purée and herbs, then mixing well.

4. Unroll the pastry and spread the tomato sauce over the top, leaving a 2.5cm (1in) gap around each edge, then sprinkle the Cheddar alternative over evenly.

5. Pinch the pastry along the longest edge and roll up as tightly as you can to form a sausage shape.

6. Cut into 1cm (½in) pieces with a sharp knife. Brush each piece all over with the beaten egg or milk alternative, then place on the prepared baking trays, leaving a 2.5cm (1in) gap between each one.

7. Bake for 18-20 minutes until golden and crispy. Cool and serve.

STORAGE
Keep covered in the fridge for up to 3 days.

Freeze for up to 3 months.

For different flavours, try adding chopped ham, sweetcorn or spinach before rolling. One of my homemade pestos (see page 104) would also make a delicious base instead of the tomato sauce.

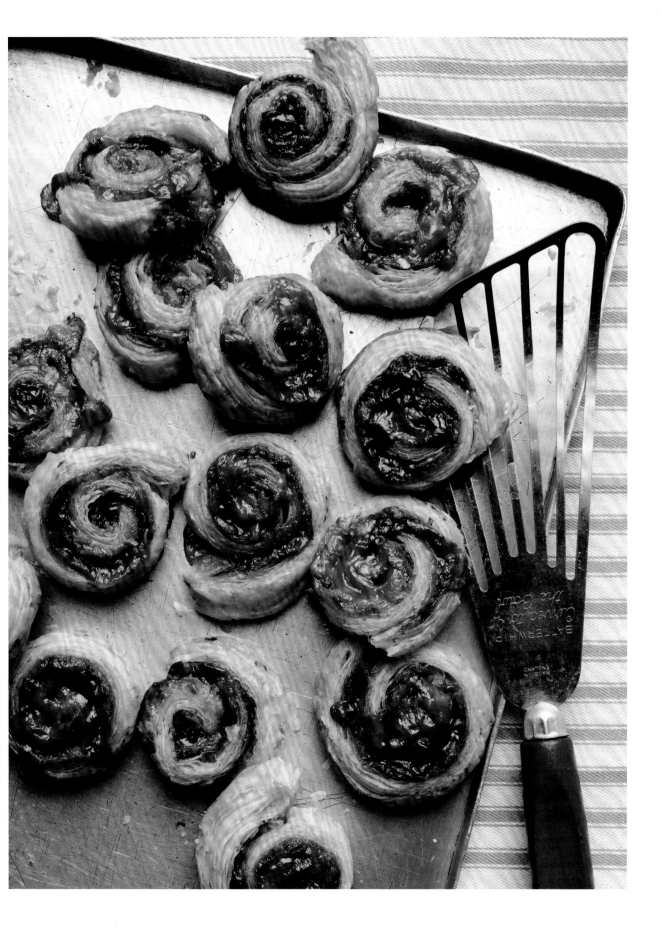

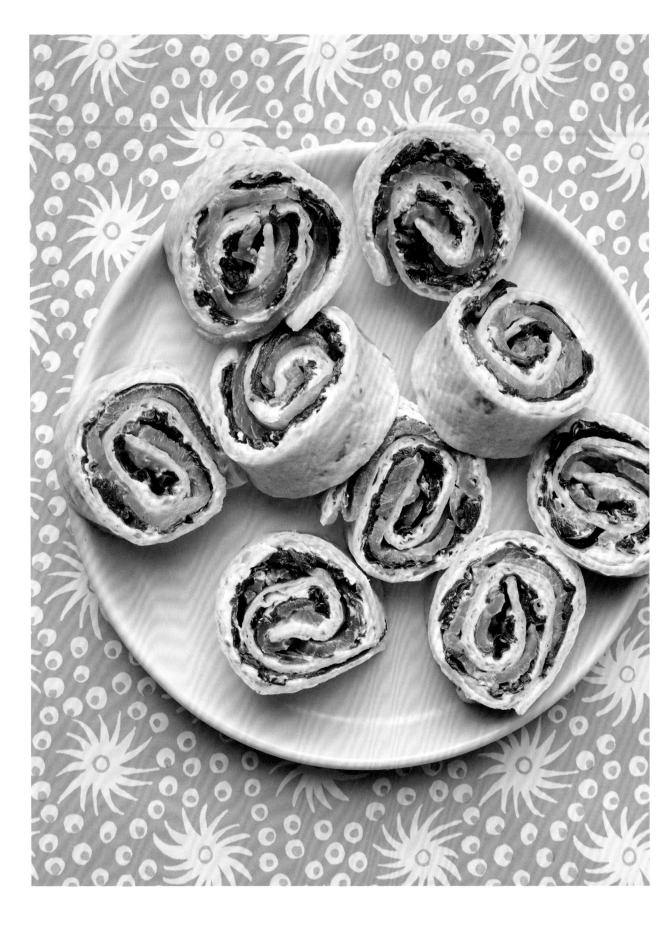

Salmon, Spinach & Soft Cheeze Spirals

Don't these tortilla roll-ups just look gorgeous? Incredibly tasty too, they're an impressive party table addition that are so quick and easy to make, but also nutritious.

EF, GF*, NF, PF, SF*, WF*

Makes: 16

Prep: 10 minutes

150g (5½oz) baby spinach leaves

3 tbsp soft cheese alternative*

2 large tortilla wraps*

80g (2¾oz) smoked salmon slices or cooked salmon flakes

1. Put the spinach leaves in a colander and pour boiling water over them until wilted. When cool, squeeze the leaves with a clean tea towel to absorb any excess water.

2. Spread the soft cheese alternative equally over the two wraps.

3. Top with a layer of spinach leaves and then the salmon.

4. For each wrap, fold over two ends and roll up tightly to make a sausage shape. Cut each wrap into 8 pieces with a sharp knife.

STORAGE
Keep covered in the fridge for up to 1 day.

Not suitable for freezing.

*Replace the salmon with diced red (bell) pepper for a veggie version.
If serving to younger babies, unroll the spirals so they can hold them in their palms.*

Carrot, Banana & Sultana Cake

This is a healthier, low-sugar take on a carrot cake, topped with a light, cream cheese-style frosting. Inspired by a recipe from an Instagram friend, Monique, I developed it into this vegan version, which was a hit at Violet's first birthday party.

EF, GF*, NF, PF, SF*, V, VG, WF*

Serves: 16–20

Prep: 30 minutes, Cook: 40 minutes

FOR THE CAKE

300g (10½oz) carrots

250g (9oz) self-raising flour* (if using gluten-free flour, add ¼ tsp xanthan gum)

1 tsp baking powder

½ tsp bicarbonate of soda

3 tsp ground cinnamon

1½ tsp ground ginger

3 small ripe bananas (approx. 350g/12oz with peel)

150ml (5fl oz) light vegetable or coconut oil, plus extra for greasing

120ml (4fl oz) plant-based milk alternative*

1½ tsp vanilla extract

4 tbsp maple syrup

110g (3¾oz) sultanas

FOR THE TOPPING

100ml (3½fl oz) whippable double cream alternative*

100g (3½oz) soft cheese alternative*

3 tbsp maple syrup

1 tsp vanilla extract

50g (1¾oz) plain Greek-style yoghurt alternative*

berries of choice

1. Preheat the oven to 190°C/Fan 170°C/375°F/Gas Mark 5 and line the base of a 20cm (8in) round cake tin with baking paper and grease the sides.

2. Peel and grate the carrots.

3. Sift the flour, baking powder and bicarbonate of soda (plus xanthan gum, if using) into a large bowl. Add the cinnamon and ginger, mix well.

4. In a separate bowl, mash the bananas, then add the oil, milk alternative, vanilla extract and maple syrup, then mix.

5. Combine the two bowls and whisk until combined, then fold in the grated carrots and the sultanas.

6. Pour the mix into the prepared cake tin, spread evenly and bake for 40–45 minutes until a skewer or knife inserted into the centre comes out clean.

7. Cool in the tin for 15 minutes, then carefully transfer to a wire rack to cool completely.

8. Meanwhile, make your frosting. Place the double cream alternative in a large bowl and whip until it forms stiff peaks.

9. In a separate bowl, add the soft cheese alternative, maple syrup, vanilla extract and Greek-style yoghurt alternative and whip until smooth. Gently fold in the whipped cream alternative until combined and refrigerate until ready to use.

10. Spread the frosting evenly over the cake, top with the berries and decorate as you wish.

STORAGE
Keep covered in the fridge for up to 3 days.

Not suitable for freezing.

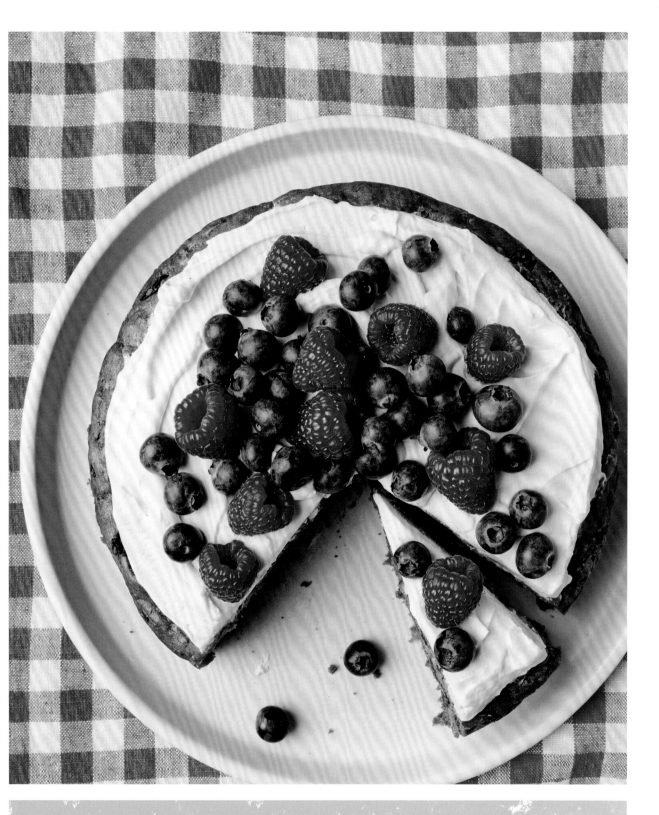

You can make the cake ahead of time, but frost and decorate just before your
event to keep as fresh as possible.

Violet's Vanilla Cupcakes

Fluffy sponge cakes with a tasty buttercream-style frosting. I had to name these after Violet because when she was born, I couldn't wait for the day we baked together, and now she's a cupcake fiend - she would happily bake and eat these every day if she had her way!

EF, GF*, NF, PF, SF*, V, VG, WF*

Makes: 12

Prep: 15 minutes, Cook: 20 minutes

FOR THE CUPCAKES

275g (9¾oz) plain flour* (*if using gluten-free flour, add ¼ tsp xanthan gum*)

2½ tsp baking powder

2½ tsp vanilla extract

4 tbsp maple syrup

250ml (9fl oz) plant-based milk alternative*

125g (4oz) butter alternative*/margarine (or 125ml/4fl oz light vegetable oil), plus extra (optional) for greasing.

FOR THE FROSTING

200g (7oz) butter alternative* or margarine*

1 tsp vanilla extract

200g (7oz) icing sugar

1. Preheat the oven to 190°C/Fan 170°C/375°F/Gas Mark 5 and line a 12-hole muffin tin with cupcake cases or grease well.

2. Sift the flour and baking powder (*plus xanthan gum, if using*) into a bowl.

3. Melt the butter alternative/margarine and add to the bowl with the vanilla extract, maple syrup and milk alternative. Whisk well for a few minutes until the batter is smooth.

4. Spoon the batter equally into the cupcake cases.

5. Bake for 20 minutes until golden, then remove from the tin and leave to cool completely on a wire rack.

6. Meanwhile, make the frosting. Cream the butter alternative or margarine, add the vanilla extract, then gradually add the icing sugar, beating together until soft and fluffy. Cool in the fridge until needed.

7. Pipe or spoon the frosting on to the cooled cupcakes.

STORAGE
Keep covered at room temperature for up to 3 days.

The cakes can be frozen (without frosting) for up to 3 months.

If using paper cupcake cases, spray some oil on them before adding the cake mixture to avoid sticking, or use silicone cupcake cases.

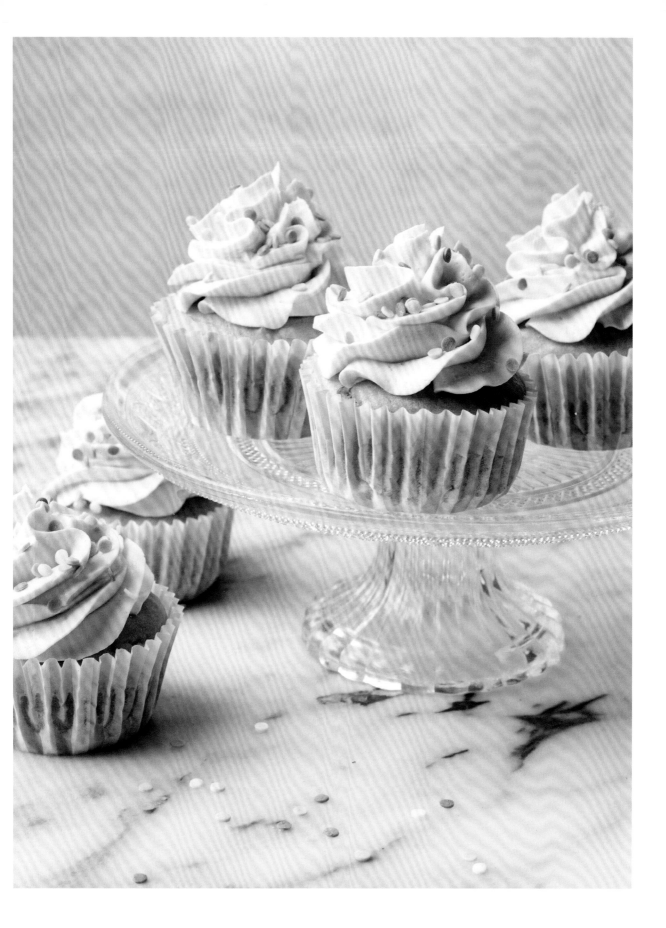

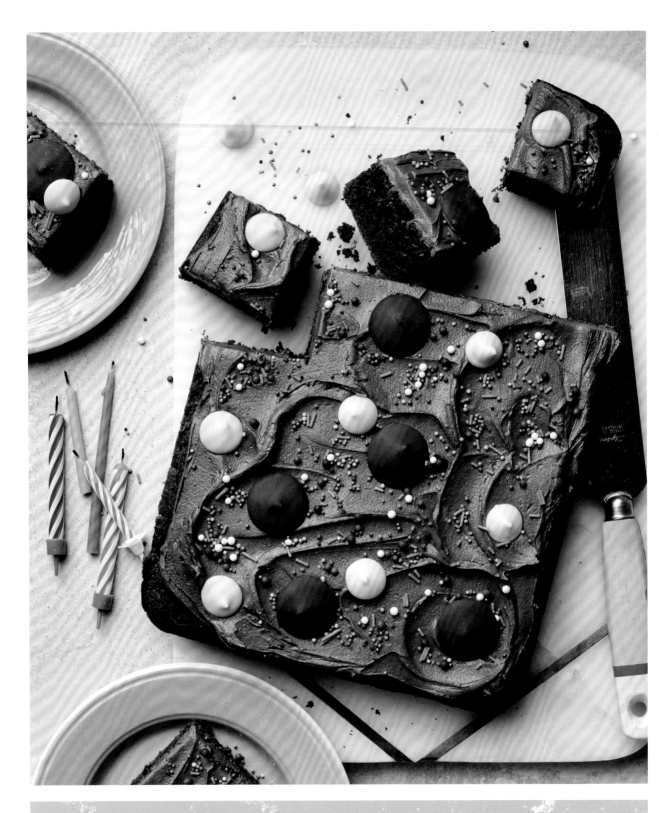

Mix up the toppings; you could try dairy-free white chocolate shavings, freeze-dried raspberries, sweeties or edible icing flowers.

Chocolate Party Traybake

Who doesn't love chocolate cake? Well this one is delicious! Rich, moist sponge with a decadent chocolate frosting and topped with treats. I'd be amazed if anyone could tell this was dairy and egg free.

EF, GF*, NF, PF, SF*, WF*, V, VG

Makes: 25 squares

Prep: 25 minutes, Cook: 30 minutes

FOR THE CAKE

300ml (10fl oz) plant-based milk alternative*

1 tbsp apple cider vinegar or lemon juice

180g (6oz) butter alternative* or margarine*

1 tsp vanilla extract

300g (10½oz) self-raising flour* (*if using gluten-free flour, add ¼ tsp xanthan gum*)

½ tsp bicarbonate of soda

4 tbsp cocoa powder

150g (5½oz) caster sugar

FOR THE CHOCOLATE FROSTING

75g (2½oz) butter alternative* or margarine*

½ tsp vanilla extract

120g (4¼oz) icing sugar

2½ tbsp cocoa powder

TOPPINGS

sugar sprinkles*

dairy-free chocolate buttons*

1. Preheat the oven to 180°C/Fan 160°C/350°F/Gas Mark 4 and line a 20cm (8in) square baking tin with baking paper.

2. In a jug, mix the milk alternative with the apple cider vinegar or lemon juice and set aside for a few minutes. This acts as a buttermilk alternative.

3. In a small pan on a low heat, melt the butter alternative or margarine, stir in the vanilla extract, then leave to cool.

4. Into a large bowl, sift the flour, bicarbonate of soda and cocoa powder (*plus xanthan gum, if using*), then add the sugar and mix well.

5. Add the milk mixture and the butter and vanilla mix, then whisk well until smooth.

6. Pour the mixture into the prepared baking tin and bake for 25–30 minutes until a skewer or knife inserted into the centre comes out clean.

7. Cool in the tin for 15 minutes, then turn out carefully on to a wire rack to cool completely.

8. Meanwhile, make your frosting. Beat together the butter alternative or margarine and vanilla extract, then gradually add the icing sugar and cocoa powder, whisking well until light and fluffy. Refrigerate until ready to use.

9. Spread evenly over the cooled cake, then sprinkle over the toppings.

STORAGE
Keep covered at room temperature for up to 3 days.

The cake can be frozen (without frosting) for up to 3 months.

Q&A

Now let's dive into the questions I get asked most by the allergy community. These answers have all been reviewed by Lucy to ensure they are based on up-to-date evidence and advice.

CMPA and other allergies

How soon should I see improvements after milk is excluded from my own or my child's diet?

It can take up to four weeks, with symptoms often improving after two weeks. Lucy says: 'It can feel frustrating not to see immediate improvements for babies with delayed CMPA, but the reality is it can often take weeks, especially if there has been a transition over to a specialist formula. It's also worth noting that for babies with immediate CMPA, symptoms should resolve more quickly.'

My baby is gaining weight, can they still have CMPA?

The short answer is yes. Both my children gained weight according to their growth chart. Faltering growth can be a symptom of CMPA but does not have to be present to confirm a diagnosis. Any concerns over weight gain should always be flagged to a healthcare professional.

Does having reflux mean a baby has CMPA?

Reflux can be a symptom of CMPA, but reflux on its own is not always indicative of allergy. Reflux is very common, affecting on average 4 out of 10 of children under a year old,[23] whereas in children with CMPA it is 1–7 out of 100. If you're concerned about reflux, do seek advice from your health visitor or GP.

Will my other children have CMPA?

This is a common concern for parents who are dealing with allergies. It is more likely that future children will also have an allergy and/or another atopic condition due to the link I previously explained (see page 17), but it isn't always the case. I know lots of parents who have one CMPA child and several allergy-free children.

Is it possible to get CMPA later in life?

It can happen as with other adult-onset allergies, but it's very rare.

Does CMPA cause reactions to beef?

You shouldn't need to avoid beef – some children react to bovine serum albumin, which is found in milk, but it's exceptionally rare. If you suspect your child reacts to beef, discuss this with your allergy team and dietitian.

Can my CMPA baby have goat's or sheep milk?

No, other mammalian milks are not suitable for children with CMPA because the proteins are very similar to cow's milk, so there is a high risk of cross-reactivity.

What happens if my child accidentally consumes dairy?

Slip ups happen more often than you'd think, especially when there's more than one child in the family who wants to share or drop their food! Take a note of what they ate, the amount and what symptoms appear. Then discuss with your dietitian. If no symptoms appear, this may be a suitable catalyst for them to start the milk ladder or start from a different step.

Can my child also react to an allergen through touch and/or airborne particles?

The vast majority of reactions occur due to ingestion (eating) the allergen. Some allergens can be airborne if vapourised when cooked (typically milk, egg and fish) but only a small percentage of children would react to exposure like this.

Can a baby get hay fever?

Hay fever (aka allergic rhinitis) is uncommon in babies and toddlers but can start in childhood and is estimated to affect around 1 in 4 people in the UK.[24] If you suspect your child may have hay fever, have a chat with a healthcare professional.

Should I go private to be seen by an allergy doctor or dietitian sooner?

Some people choose to pay privately (or claim through private medical insurance) to be seen quicker than their local NHS waiting list. You can expect a consultation with a private paediatric allergy doctor to cost hundreds of pounds, with allergy tests often costing extra. The decision to do this is entirely personal, but my advice would be to make sure you have a clear objective in mind as to what you want to get out of the appointment if you're spending a significant amount of money on it. For example, is it testing you'd like (which remember, won't be useful for children with non-IgE mediated CMPA), a diagnosis or general advice? Then assess the financials and make the right decision for you.

If I'm soya free, do I need to avoid soya lecithin?

Soya lecithin is an emulsifier, which is often used to mix ingredients together and stop them separating, or to improve the texture of the product. Some products use soya-free emulsifiers such as sunflower. Soya lecithin contains very little soya protein, and many children are able to tolerate it without concern. As always with allergy, this can be child dependent, so have a chat with your healthcare professional, who may also guide on how to trial the introduction of it.

If tolerated, it opens up many more food choices. It's also worth mentioning that refined soya oil will not be labelled on packs where it's used, because the product is so heavily refined that the allergy-causing proteins are removed.

My child is allergic to peanuts, do they have to avoid all nuts?

Peanuts are technically a legume (like a pea!), rather than a tree nut. Those with an existing peanut allergy have an increased likelihood of around 30–40% of developing a tree nut allergy,[25] so you may be advised to have IgE testing for some or all tree nuts to guide on which are safe to consume. The general advice would be to continue consuming nuts that they aren't allergic to in order to maintain tolerance, however, there are risks of cross-contamination in products with nuts as an ingredient, so this is always best to discuss with your healthcare professional.

If my baby reacts to wheat, do I need to avoid all gluten?

It's important to remember the difference between wheat and gluten (see page 50). Children who have a wheat allergy may be reacting to any of the key proteins in wheat, which may or may not include gluten. Your healthcare professional may suggest trialling a wheat-free diet initially (but without exclusion of gluten in other foods, e.g. rye/barley), or avoidance of gluten too. For children with coeliac disease, they will need to exclude all foods containing gluten, including rye and barley.

What is immunotherapy and can it cure allergies?

Immunotherapy (also called desensitisation) is a treatment that aims to desensitise your immune system to the food you are allergic to, meaning you're less likely to have a reaction. It does this by gradually exposing you to small amounts of that food under careful supervision, slowly building up the amounts over the weeks and months. The goal of the treatment is to stop you having an allergic reaction if you accidentally come into contact with the food that you are allergic to. It's not a cure for allergy, but in some cases, treatment can be so successful that you can go on to freely eat the food. Immunotherapy for food allergies has been getting more press attention recently, and it does offer a glimmer of hope for allergy parents that this could be used more widely in the future. Palforzia was approved by the NHS in 2021 to treat certain children aged 4–17 with peanut allergies, and some specialist NHS clinic trials now offer oral immunotherapy for older children with more serious or persistent egg or milk allergies. Clinical trials are underway for further use of immunotherapy treatments in regard to allergies. For more information about immunotherapy, there is a factsheet available on the Anaphylaxis UK website.[26]

The milk ladder

My child has several allergies, how do I approach ladders?

You should definitely push for dietitian support if dealing with more than one allergy. It's important to only attempt one ladder at a time, to be able to pinpoint reactions. Lucy says: 'When faced with multiple ladders parents often ask me, "Which one first?". There is no rule here, and often we discuss which one will help liberalise a child's diet most at home and in childcare, for example. You can also move between ladders, e.g. focus on the baked steps of the milk ladder, then pause that ladder and move over to the baked steps of the egg ladder, returning to the milk ladder and so on.'

If I'm breastfeeding, do I need to complete the milk ladder first before my child?

The milk ladder was formulated with direct reintroduction to the allergic child in mind – for a breastfeeding mum it's generally recommended to reintroduce dairy back into your diet in what would be considered 'normal' amounts (2-4 portions a day across a week) and then monitor for any symptoms prior to starting the milk ladder with your child. However, if this makes you feel anxious, you can start the ladder with your child first, then introduce any steps that are tolerated back into your diet.

What if my child refuses the food on a milk ladder step?

This is so common! Try to get creative and mix with something else – so instead of a whole biscuit, you could crumble it on to dairy-free yoghurt. Or for a muffin, spread some jam on to it. If they are not accepting your disguise attempts, speak to your dietitian or if you are dealing with a mild allergy, you may consider moving to a small portion of the next step and monitoring for reactions.

For more information on the milk ladder see page 28.

Nutrition and supplements

Is it true that soya should be avoided by boys?
No. Stories circulated on the internet previously claiming that eating soya affects hormone levels in males and could lead to fertility issues, but there is no robust evidence to support this. Soya contains isoflavones which are a type of phytoestrogen. This has some structural similarities to oestrogen but when ingested into the body it behaves differently. Soya is considered safe for consumption in the UK from 6 months+ for both boys and girls and research points to health benefits associated with regular soya consumption, including reduced risk of certain cancers and cardiovascular benefits.

What is a 'portion' for a child when considering the healthy eating guidelines?
It may be smaller than you think! A general guide for fruit and veg, for example, is that a portion is what would fit into the palm of your child's hand, e.g. ½ banana or apple, 3 large strawberries, 3 florets of broccoli, 1½ tablespoons peas, carrots or sweetcorn or 1 slice of melon.

Should I be worried about the salt and sugar in plant-based milk?
It's definitely one to be aware of, as there aren't currently any fortified PBMAs on the market that don't contain salt and/or sugars. Be aware that the salt in PBMA will count towards your child's daily salt limits, so it's even more important to ensure that their food doesn't contain added salt. While there are natural sugars in cow's milk (from lactose), in PBMAs there can be added sugars, which can contribute to tooth decay, so it's best to choose unsweetened ones where possible.

Can you get calcium supplements for babies?
Not typically, as the best way for your child to get their calcium requirements is through a healthy diet and fortified PBMA. It is possible to meet your child's calcium requirements with ease on a milk-free diet; see page 34. There are multivitamins with added calcium available from 3 years+.

Should I be giving my child a probiotic?
Probiotics are a supplement that contain good bacteria which, when given in the right amounts, can provide a health benefit to you/your child. If you're breastfeeding, your breast milk naturally contains probiotics and prebiotics (e.g. human milk oligosaccharides... oof that's a long word!), and some hypoallergenic formula does include pre- and/or probiotics, but this isn't a requirement under UK law. They are considered safe for children, but scientific studies remain ongoing with regard to potential benefits, including for children with or at risk of food allergies. There is some robust evidence to support the use of certain probiotic strains with certain conditions, including colic and antibiotic-associated diarrhoea. I'd always suggest discussing this with a dietitian or healthcare professional.

Labels

My child is allergic to an uncommon allergen, how will I find this on the labels?

Any allergens outside of the top 14 won't be highlighted in bold on the pack, but should always be listed in the ingredient list, so you'll need to read the full list on every pack you buy.

Why are pine nuts not labelled in bold on packs?

Pine nuts are not actually tree nuts, but a seed. So they don't fit into the top 14 allergens which require labelling in the UK (see page 50). It is possible to be allergic to pine nuts, so if you suspect that you/or your child are, please discuss it with your GP or dietitian.

If I notice the allergy labelling on a pack, or in an establishment is incorrect, what should I do?

If you're in a restaurant or food business, firstly communicate this to the manager, then report it via your nearest Trading Standards office.

Weaning

Is food before one just for fun?

There's no doubt you'll hear this saying bandied about! It basically comes from a point of trying to reassure parents by suggesting that before one year of age children don't really need solid food as they're getting their nutrition from milk. However, the phrase isn't correct! While milk will still be the primary source of nutrition, solid food is important to boost nutrients, especially iron, as baby's iron stores run out at six months. Eating solid food is also important for a baby's development and for them to accept new flavours and textures. Also, as I've mentioned, introducing allergens is important before the age of one to help reduce the likelihood of allergies. So, should it be fun? Yes. But just for fun? No.

If I'm vegan, do I still need to introduce fish/seafood as an allergen?

This is a personal choice. Generally the guidance is that you only need to introduce foods that you continue to consume in your diet, as repeated exposure maintains tolerance. However, you may want to be aware of any potential allergies, to avoid an unexpected reaction should your child happen to consume something containing that allergen. You should also consider that there is a risk (which is currently difficult to quantify as research is limited) that if it isn't maintained in the diet then an allergy could potentially develop.

How much milk should my child be drinking?

If breastfeeding, babies will naturally reduce their milk intake as they increase solid food consumption. For formula-fed babies, the NHS guidance for 6-12 months old is around 500-600ml (18-20fl oz) per day, and around 300-400ml (10-14fl oz) per day from age 1+.

Key Nutrient Information

In this table you'll find a summary of key nutrients (important for everyone, not just those on a dairy-free diet), including the daily requirements per age, based on the current UK government recommendations.[27] Also included are good dairy-free sources for each nutrient, so this can be used as a cheat sheet to make sure you're regularly including a range of these in yours and your child's diet.

MACRONUTRIENTS

Nutrient	Why it's required	Daily requirements (mg = milligrams, mcg = micrograms)	Good dairy-free sources
STARCHY CARBOHYDRATES (ENERGY)	Gives the body readily available energy, important vitamins and fibre.	This can vary by size and other factors, so see 'a healthy balanced diet' on page 35. Many carbohydrate foods contain fibre, which is very filling and babies only need in small amounts. If a large amount of fibre is eaten, their tummies can get full quickly and they wouldn't have the opportunity to get nutrients from other foods.	Potatoes Pasta, rice and grains (couscous, bulgur wheat) Bread Oats
PROTEIN	Helps the body grow and repair itself, especially the muscles and bones.	Age 1-3: 14.5g Age 4-6: 19.7g Age 7-10: 28.3g Age 11-14: 42.1g (males); 41.2g (females) Age 15-18: 55.2g (males); 45g (females) Age 19-64: 55.5g (males); 45g (females) Age 65+: 53.3g (males); 46.5g (females) Pregnancy: requirements above +6g Breastfeeding: requirements above +11g when baby is 0-6 months +8g when baby is 6 months+	Eggs Fish Meat Legumes, e.g. beans, lentils and chickpeas Nuts/nut butter Seeds, e.g. chia, flax, sunflower, pumpkin Quinoa Soya products, e.g. tofu, tempeh, soya milk and yoghurt alternatives
FATS	Provide the body with energy and essential fatty acids (omega-3 and omega-6). Help absorption of vitamins A, D, E and K.	Some fat is needed, but you should aim for healthy fats shown here. It's important not to have too much saturated fat, which is found in processed foods such as biscuits and cakes.	**Omega-3** Oily fish, e.g. salmon, sardines, mackerel Seeds, e.g. flax and chia **Omega-6** Nuts, seeds, vegetable oils, margarine Other fat sources: Oils (olive, coconut, vegetable, sunflower) Avocado Olives

MICRONUTRIENTS

Nutrient	Why it's required	Daily requirements (mg = milligrams, mcg = micrograms)	Good dairy-free sources
CALCIUM	To maintain strong bones and teeth, plus healthy muscle and nerve function.	Under 1: 525mg Age 1-3: 350mg Age 4-6: 450mg Age 7-10: 550mg Age 11-18 females: 800mg Age 11-18 males: 1,000mg Adults: 700mg When breastfeeding: 1,250mg	Calcium-fortified plant-based milk, yoghurt and cheese alternatives* Calcium-fortified breakfast cereals* Bread (fortified with calcium by UK law) Calcium-set tofu (N.B. contains soya) Canned fish with soft bones, e.g. sardines, pilchards, salmon Oranges White beans Chia seeds Green leafy veg (spring greens, broccoli, bok choy)
IODINE	For production of thyroid hormones which regulate metabolic rate, growth and development. During pregnancy, infancy, and early childhood it also supports development of baby's brain.	Age 1-3: 70mcg Age 4-6: 100mcg Age 7-10: 110mcg Age 11-14: 130mcg Adults and 15+: 140mcg In pregnancy: 200mcg When breastfeeding: 250mcg[28]	White fish, e.g. cod, haddock, basa Shellfish, e.g. prawns Eggs Iodine-fortified plant-based milk and yoghurt alternatives* Seaweed (but should be avoided in young children) Sources with lower amounts: oily fish, e.g. salmon, and canned tuna
IRON	Important for making haemoglobin, a substance in red blood cells, which transports oxygen around the body.	Babies are born with iron stores which last until they are around six months old, so iron is an important nutrient to consider from that point (although breastmilk and formula both contribute to iron requirements). 7-12 months: 7.8mg Age 1-3: 6.9mg Age 4-6: 6.1mg Age 7-10: 8.7mg Age 11-18: 11.3mg (males); 14.8mg (females) Age 19-49: 8.7mg (males); 14.8mg (females) Age 50+: 8.7mg (males), 8.7mg (females post-menopause) Side effects are possible from consuming high doses of iron (over 20mg).	**Haem sources** (absorbed more easily): Red meat Offal Fish (especially oily fish) Poultry **Non-haem sources** (absorbed less easily, but eating alongside a vitamin C source aids absorption) Eggs Legumes, e.g. beans, chickpeas, lentils Dark green vegetables, e.g. spinach, kale, broccoli Nuts and seeds Fortified products,* e.g. white bread, breakfast cereals

Nutrient	Why it's required	Daily requirements (mg = milligrams, mcg = micrograms)	Good dairy-free sources
VITAMIN A (Retinol)	Helps the immune system work properly, defending against illness and infection. Keeps skin healthy. Helps vision in dim light.	Age 1-6: 400mcg Age 7-10: 500mcg Age 11-14: 600mcg Adults and 15+: 700mcg (males); 600mcg (females) Too much vitamin A when pregnant can harm your unborn baby so avoid vitamin A supplements and liver products.	Eggs Oily fish Fortified products* Liver (avoid when pregnant, and moderate amounts in young children) You can also get vitamin A by including good sources of beta-carotene in your diet, as the body can convert this into retinol: yellow, red, and green (leafy) vegetables, e.g. spinach, carrots, sweet potatoes, red peppers, yellow fruit, e.g. mango, papaya, apricots
VITAMIN B2 (Riboflavin)	Helps the body to release energy from food. Keeps the skin, eyes and nervous system healthy.	Age 1-3: 0.6mg Age 4-6: 0.8mg Age 7-10: 1mg Age 11-14: 1.2mg (males); 1.1mg (females) Adults and 15+: 1.3mg (males); 1.1mg (females)	Fortified plant-based milk alternatives* Eggs Fortified breakfast cereal* Mushrooms
VITAMIN B12	Supports normal function of nerve cells, blood cell formation and DNA synthesis. Needed to prevent megaloblastic anaemia which can cause extreme tiredness.	Age 1-3: 0.5mcg Age 4-6: 0.8mcg Age 7-10: 1mcg Age 11-14: 1.2mcg Adults and 15+: 1.5mcg	Beef Pork Poultry Eggs Fish Fortified products*, e.g. plant-based milk, yoghurt alternatives, Marmite®, nutritional yeast, breakfast cereal
VITAMIN C	Helps to protect cells and keep them healthy. Supports immune system. Forms collagen, which maintains healthy skin, blood vessels and bones. Helps absorption of non-haem iron.	Age 1-10: 30mg Age 11-14: 35mg Adults and 15+: 40mg	Citrus fruits, e.g. oranges, lemons, limes Kiwi fruit Bell peppers Tomatoes Broccoli Strawberries Blackcurrants Potatoes Kale Brussels sprouts

Nutrient	Why it's required	Daily requirements (mg = milligrams, mcg = micrograms)	Good dairy-free sources
VITAMIN D	Helps absorption of calcium and phosphate into the body to maintain strong bones, muscles and teeth.	10mcg See advice on supplements on page 36.	Sunlight Eggs Red meat Offal Oily fish Mushrooms Fortified products,* e.g. plant-based milk, margarine and yoghurt alternatives
ZINC	Important for immune function, growth and development.	Age 1-3: 5mg Age 4-6: 6.5mg Age 7-10: 7mg Age 11-14: 9mg Age 15+: 9.5mg (males); 7mg (females)	Meat Shellfish and other seafood Legumes e.g. beans, lentils and chickpeas Nuts and seeds

* Not all plant-based products are fortified, so you'll need to check packs for details of the individual nutrient fortification.

FURTHER READING

Don't forget to check out my Instagram page **@thedairyfreemum** and website **www.thedairyfreemum.com** for lots more tips and tricks. Here's a selection of other websites I'd recommend for further reading. Many have downloadable fact sheets which can be helpful to send to family and friends.

Websites

Allergy UK - Excellent information about allergies, handy factsheets and even a helpline: **www.allergyuk.org** IG: @allergy_uk

Anaphylaxis UK - Lots of helpful information and support materials for those at risk of anaphylaxis: **www.anaphylaxis.org.uk** IG: @anaphylaxisuk

BSACI (The British Society for Allergy and Clinical Immunology) - Check out the patients tab and resources including Allergy Action Plan templates: **www.bsaci.org**

Beat Asthma - Resources for children and young people with asthma: **www.beatasthma.co.uk**

British Red Cross - In the First Aid section there are lots of guides and accompanying videos for various paediatric illnesses and emergency situations: **www.redcross.org.uk** IG: @britishredcross

Coeliac UK - Essential information, tips and research into coeliac disease: **www.coeliac.org.uk** IG: @coeliacuk

FPIES (Food Protein Induced Enterocolitis Syndrome) UK - Support and advice for families affected by FPIES: www.fpiesuk.org

Food Standards Agency (FSA) - Guidance for food businesses on providing allergen information and a sign-up service for allergy alerts: **www.food.gov.uk/allergy** IG: @foodgov

National Eczema Society - Information for everyone impacted by eczema, with helpful booklets and a helpline: **www.eczema.org** IG: @eczemasociety

NHS - Comprehensive advice for an A-Z of health concerns: **www.nhs.uk** IG: @nhs

The Allergy Team - Information, support and training for families, schools and businesses to help manage food allergies: **www.theallergyteam.com** IG: @theallergyteam

The Natasha Allergy Research Foundation - A charity leading pioneering research and campaigning for allergy awareness: **www.narf.org.uk** IG: @natashasfoundation

Instagram Pages

As my community has been built through Instagram, I also wanted to include some of my favourite accounts for you to follow. It's so amazing to see the incredible information available on social media now, just make sure this never replaces personalised medical advice.

@childrensdietitian - Lucy Upton's page is full of incredibly helpful info on allergies, weaning, feeding and nutrition (as well as being the wonderful dietitian for this book!).

@dradamfox - Professor Adam Fox is a leading specialist paediatric allergy doctor sharing posts and videos discussing key allergy topics.

@drhelenallergy - Dr Helen Evans-Howells is a GP, allergy mum and allergy lecturer. Also check out her Facebook group for amazing info and support.

@feedeatspeak - Stacey Zimmels focuses on support for breastfeeding, bottle feeding, weaning and fussy eating.

@foodsafetymum - Jenna Brown is a food safety expert and shares info and tips for storing and cooking food safely.

@solidstarts - Solid Starts are a team of paediatric feeding therapists, doctors and dietitians sharing advice for introducing solids, including helpful visuals of how to prepare first foods.

@sr_nutrition - Charlotte Stirling-Reed is a true weaning expert; her page is packed full of tips and her books are also excellent.

@theallergydietitian - Dr Penny Barnard is a paediatric dietitian with a wealth of experience and shares really helpful info.

@drstephanieooi - Dr Stephanie Jen Chyi Ooi is a GP and allergy mum; she shares informative posts about various health topics.

@themilkallergydietitian - Lydia Collins-Hussey is a paediatric allergy dietitian who posts specifically about CMPA; she also happened to be Violet's dietitian!

GLOSSARY

AAI Adrenaline Auto-Injector, a device prescribed to people who are at risk of anaphylaxis.

Allergy Action Plan Medical plans completed by a healthcare professional for children at risk of anaphylaxis, with instructions for what to do in an emergency.

Allergy Focused Clinical History A series of questions used by a healthcare professional as the key first step in allergy diagnosis and to decide which tests should be undertaken.

Anaphylaxis A severe, life-threatening allergic reaction, to a food, medicine or insect sting to which the body is hypersensitive. Read more on page 54.

Antibody A protective protein produced by the immune system in response to a substance that your body perceives as harmful.

Antihistamines A type of medication used to neutralise the effects of histamine (released during an allergic response) or to inhibit its production in the body. Widely used to help relieve certain allergy symptoms.

Atopy The genetic tendency to develop an atopic condition.

Atopic Condition Relating to allergy, asthma, hay fever and/ or eczema.

Healthcare Professional A person contracted to provide a healthcare service to a patient, including doctors, nurses, midwives, health visitors, dietitians, paramedics, clinical psychologists and pharmacists.

Histamine A chemical found in some cells in the body, which is released into the bloodstream when your body comes into contact with a substance you are allergic to. Histamine is what makes your body produce allergic symptoms.

Hives (or Urticaria) An itchy rash with raised bumps or patches on the skin.

IgE Mediated An immediate-type allergy with symptoms presenting within minutes and up to two hours after ingesting the allergen.

Immune System The body's defence tool to protect, prevent or limit infection.

Immunoglobulin E (IgE) The type of antibody released by the body in an immediate-type allergic reaction.

Immunotherapy A medical treatment that aims to desensitise your immune system to the food you are allergic to, meaning you're less likely to have a reaction. Read more on page 206.

Isoflavones A class of phytoestrogens produced mainly by plants of the legume family, especially soya beans.

Lancet A small, pointed surgical instrument, usually two-edged, used for skin prick tests (see page 24).

Non-IgE Mediated A delayed-type allergy with symptoms presenting from two hours up to 72 hours after ingesting the allergen.

Nutrient A substance that provides nourishment essential for people to live and grow.

Paediatric Allergy Dietitian A registered and qualified dietitian who works with children and their families to help them with nutrition, growth and practical aspects of managing food allergies.

Phytoestrogen Substances that occur naturally in plants that have a similar chemical structure to the female hormone oestrogen.

PBMA Plant-Based Milk Alternative.

Wheal (or Welt) An individual hive, measured on the skin during skin prick allergy tests (see page 24).

REFERENCES

[1] Al-Beltagi, M., Saeed, N,K., Bediwy, A.S., Elbeltagi R., 'Cow's milk-induced gastrointestinal disorders: From infancy to adulthood', *World J Clin Pediatr*. 2022 Nov 9;11(6):437-454. doi: 10.5409/wjcp.v11.i6.437. PMID: 36439902; PMCID: PMC9685681

[2] Luyt, D., Ball, H., Makwana, N., Green, M.R., Bravin, K., Nasser, S.M., Clark, A.T., 'Standards of Care Committee (SOCC) of the British Society for Allergy and Clinical Immunology (BSACI). BSACI guideline for the diagnosis and management of cow's milk allergy', *Clin Exp Allergy*. 2014;44(5):642-72. doi: 10.1111/cea.12302. PMID: 24588904

[3] Schoemaker, A.A., Sprikkelman, A.B., Grimshaw, K.E., Roberts, G., Grabenhenrich, L., Rosenfeld, L., Siegert, S., Dubakiene, R., Rudzeviciene, O., Reche, M., Fiandor, A., Papadopoulos, N.G., Malamitsi-Puchner, A., Fiocchi, A., Dahdah, L., Sigurdardottir, S.T., Clausen, M., Stańczyk-Przyłuska, A., Zeman, K., Mills, E.N., McBride, D., Keil, T., Beyer, K., 'Incidence and natural history of challenge-proven cow's milk allergy in European children--EuroPrevall birth cohort', *Allergy*. 2015 Aug;70(8):963-72. doi: 10.1111/all.12630. Epub 2015 May 18. PMID: 25864712

[4] https://www.nhs.uk/conditions/food-allergy/

[5] Ludman, S., Shah, N., Fox, A.T., 'Managing Cow's Milk Allergy in Children', *BMJ*. 2013; 347:f5424

[6] National Eczema Society: our skin & eczema

[7] Allergy UK, Impact Report 2012

[8] https://gpifn.files.wordpress.com/2019/10/imap_final_ladder-may_2017_original.pdf

[9] https://gpifn.files.wordpress.com/2019/10/imap-recipes_final_original.pdf

[10] BDA UK Healthy eating for children –https://www.bda.uk.com/resourceLibrary/printPdf/?resource=healthy-eating-for-children

[11] NHS 'Do I need vitamin supplements?' https://www.nhs.uk/common-health-questions/food-and-diet/do-i-need-vitamin-supplements/

[12] Recommended by BDA following WHO recommendations

[13] https://www.who.int/news-room/fact-sheets/detail/infant-and-young-child-feeding

[14] Vandenplas, Y., Koletzko, S., Isolauri, E., Hill, D., Oranje, A.P., Brueton, M., Staiano, A., Dupont, C., 'Guidelines for the diagnosis and management of cow's milk protein allergy in infants', Arch Dis Child. 2007 Oct;92(10):902–8. doi: 10.1136/adc.2006.110999. Erratum in: *Arch Dis Child*. 2007 Oct;92(10):following 908. Erratum in: Arch Dis Child. 2008 Jan;93(1):93. PMID: 17895338; PMCID: PMC2083222

[15] NHS Sussex Health & Care Partnership – guidance for prescribing cow's milk allergy formula, 2022

[16] BSACI – Infant feeding and allergy prevention, guidance for parents, 2018

[17] https://www.keepabeat.com/

[18] Ierodiakonou, D., Garcia-Larsen, V., Logan, A., et al., 'Timing of Allergenic Food Introduction to the Infant Diet and Risk of Allergic or Autoimmune Disease: A Systematic Review and Meta-analysis', *JAMA*. 2016;316(11):1181–1192. doi:10.1001/jama.2016.12623

[19] Allergy UK, Weaning Your Food Allergenic Baby

[20] https://yellowcard.mhra.gov.uk/

[21] https://www.bsaci.org/professional-resources/resources/paediatric-allergy-action-plans/

[22] Government Department of Education – Keeping Children Safe in Education 2023

[23] NICE guideline – Gastro-oesophageal reflux disease in children and young people: diagnosis and management, 2015

[24] Scadding, G.K., Kariyawasam, H.H., Scadding, G., Mirakian, R., Buckley, R.J., Dixon, T., Durham, S.R., Farooque, S., Jones, N., Leech, S., Nasser, S.M., Powell, R., Roberts, G., Rotiroti, G., Simpson, A., Smith, H., Clark, A.T., 'BSACI guideline for the diagnosis and management of allergic and non-allergic rhinitis' (Revised Edition 2017; First edition 2007). *Clin Exp Allergy*. 2017 Jul;47(7):856–889. doi: 10.1111/cea.12953. PMID: 30239057

[25] Allergy UK Tree Nut Allergy Factsheet 2022

[26] https://www.anaphylaxis.org.uk/wp-content/uploads/2023/08/Food-Immunotherapy-V4.pdf

[27] UK requirements as per the Government Dietary Recommendations 2016 – https://assets.publishing.service.gov.uk/media/5a749fece5274a44083b82d8/government_dietary_recommendations.pdf

[28] Based on WHO requirements as recommended by the BDA

ACKNOWLEDGEMENTS

Firstly, I want to say a huge thank you to anyone who has followed and supported @thedairyfreemum on Instagram over the years. You've made this all possible, giving me the chance to call something I'm so passionate about my 'job'. The allergy parent community is so supportive, and I'm so grateful to each and every one of you.

To Violet and Jude - my inspirations, and my greatest achievements. I wish you hadn't had to go through so much with allergies and health issues at such at a young age, but goodness I am so proud of your resilience. Thank you for being my chief recipe testers and harshest critics, for the cuddles, laughter and unwavering love. This book is for you.

Mike, your incredible support along the way has meant so much, from taking the kids out every weekend so I can be writing and cooking, to sharing my excitement and giving me a boost when I struggled. Thank you.

To my wonderful family, particularly Mum (promise I've forgiven you for the eggs!), Dad, Olga, Paul, Jamie, Ben, and all my extended family in Canada.

This book's journey all began with Lauren, my amazing agent, and fellow allergy mum. Thank you for making my dreams come true! The moment I first received a message from you will always be imprinted in my mind as one of the most exciting of my life.

To the wonderful team at Yellow Kite - thank you for believing in me. Nicky and Liv, I knew I'd found the right team at our first meeting - your passion for why this book is so important for allergy parents shone through (cemented by the dairy-free biscuits!) You've been so supportive, kind, and made this journey fun, collaborative and rewarding.

I'm so grateful to the incredible team who have helped to bring this book to life. To Jen for the stunning photos, you captured how I wanted the food to look perfectly. Louise for your creative vision and the gorgeous design of the pages. Vicky for your fantastic copy editing, and the many more people involved behind the scenes.

Lucy, thank you not only for your exceptional work as paediatric dietitian on this book (your knowledge and understanding is second to none!) but also for your support since the early days of my page. A big thanks also to the other wonderful dietitians, nutritionists and healthcare professionals who I've learned so much from throughout this journey, in particular Lydia, Paula, Charlotte SR, Penny and Helen.

To my lovely friends, thank you for your advice and support throughout. Shout-out to Eleanor for making my nails look pretty and the many supportive chats, and Liv for always making my recipes despite not being dairy free! Also to #Charlotte @sr_nutrition and Sophie @thefoldinglady for your kind testimonials in the initial proposal.

All that's left is for me to say how hopeful I am that you've found this book helpful, and that you love the recipes. I can't wait to see your creations.

INDEX

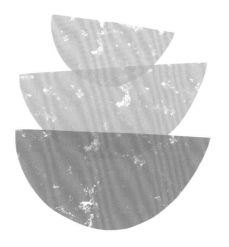

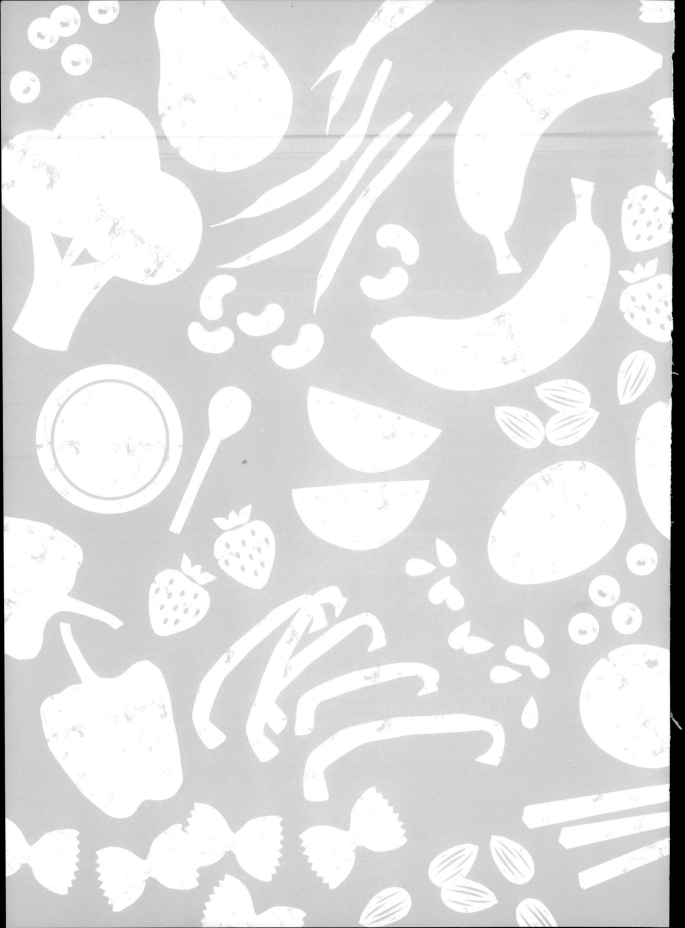